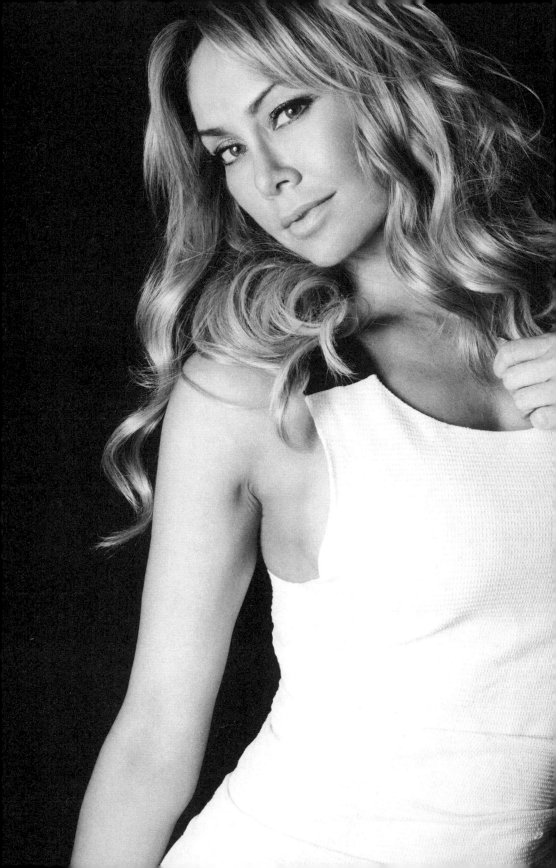

To my Mum:
Thank you for being there every step of the way. I would
not be where I am today without your love and support.
I love you.

To Robert, who encouraged me to write this book and
makes me believe every day that anything is possible.

THE 5678 Diet

The 14-Day Plan for Healthy, Lasting Weight Loss

KYM JOHNSON

with Karen Moline

Regan Arts.

New York

Regan Arts.

65 Bleecker Street
New York, NY 10012

First Regan Arts hardcover edition, January 2016.

Library of Congress Control Number: 2015951637

ISBN 978-1-942872-91-7

Interior design by Nancy Singer
Jacket design by Richard Ljoenes
Jacket photograph by Glenn Nutley
Interior photographs: Glenn Nutley, iv, 34, 36, 52, 80, 98, 126, 128, 156, 216, 228, 258, 260, 288, 302; Courtesy of the author, vi, 7, 10, 149, 286; Adam Taylor/Getty Images, x, 292; Lesley Bryce, xii, 161–215, 231–257; Henry S. Dziekan III/Getty Images, 2; Craig Sjodin/Getty Images, 32.

Printed in the United States of America

10 9 8 7 6 5 4 3 2 1

CONTENTS

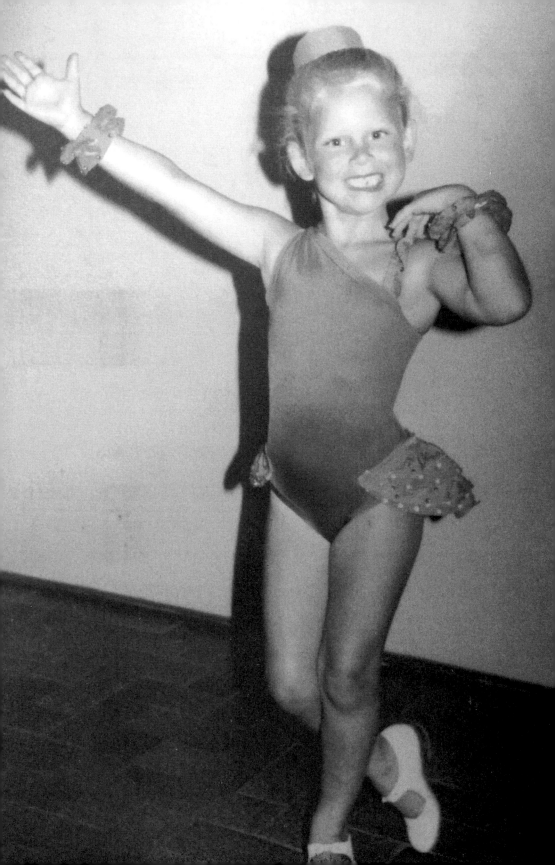

Introduction

I can't remember my world without dancing in it.

I started dancing when I was three and loved it from the first minute I set foot in the studio. My mum had been a dancer herself, and she recognized and nurtured my potential early on, letting me take jazz, tap, ballet, and music theater classes after school and on weekends. On days when I didn't have dance classes I would come home and practice my dancing before *The Brady Bunch* came on the telly. On Saturdays, I'd be at the Langshores Dance Studio in Sydney from ten in the morning till three or four in the afternoon, but I didn't mind at all. I loved to dance, and the girls in the class were my best friends. Often they'd come over to my house afterward and we'd watch *Annie* and tell ourselves we'd be stars someday.

Because that's what people see when they look at dancers—stars. They see the beautiful costumes, the bright smiles, the effortless grace. But dancing's not as easy as it looks, especially for women. We dance in three-and-a-half-inch heels and need to be highly flexible, doing splits, being lifted and thrown around. I actually can't believe I'm still dancing at my age, up against colleagues who are a generation younger than I am!

I often say that I've been lucky enough to have a career doing what I love for my whole adult life. But then I realize that's not quite true. Yes, there was quite a bit of luck involved, but luck has little to do with hard work. And I mean hard, hard work. My days have been filled with dance classes since I was a very little girl, and it was hard work to get to them and stand in front of those mirrors and rehearse and practice and rehearse some more even when my feet were screaming at me to stop and my teacher's frown told me that I wasn't even close to mastering the routine.

Like all professional athletes, dancers are a particular breed. Our careers are finite. We run the risk of an injury that could stop us in our tracks every time we rehearse or perform. We work in a highly competitive world where we are always being judged and reminded that someone else is better, or taller, or more shapely, or stronger, or more flexible . . . you get the point.

So why do we dance? That's easy. Because we love it.

And this love makes everything worthwhile. It sustained me whenever I had an off day and performed poorly in a competition and wondered if I'd ever do better again. It sustained me when tours were canceled, when the jobs I thought I had evaporated overnight. It sustained me through my parents' divorce. It sustained me even when I had a broken heart.

When you love what you do, it's not a chore. It's one of the greatest gifts you can have. So even if circumstances have left you feeling stuck or frustrated at the moment, finding something you truly love and working toward making that love a reality should be one of your top priorities. I never dreamed I would be a two-time Mirror Ball winner. I never dreamed I would meet a man like Robert Herjavec, an incredibly successful businessman and entrepreneur, whom you might know from ABC's *Shark Tank*— or as my partner on the tenth-anniversary season of *Dancing with the Stars*. But dreams can come true—they just take a little work. Trust me on this!

●●●●

What makes a dancer? A natural sense of rhythm and love for music and movement, of course. A sense of grace. A love of performing. A fierce inner motivation and drive. Knowing when to start, and knowing when to stop. And a willingness to work hard and keep at it, with discipline and determination, until we get it right.

In other words, dancing teaches you how to be a winner. Not in the classic sense of coming in first or being on top, but a true winner, someone who works hard, follows their dreams, and is gracious even in defeat. I've been so blessed for my entire run on *Dancing with the Stars*. I won the ninth season with Donny Osmond and the twelfth with Super Bowl champ wide receiver Hines Ward, and I was even invited back to judge on the Australian version of the show. But while I'm proud of these successes, I know they don't define me. Rejection is a part of life, and what matters is your resilience. How do you cope with obstacles in your way? How do you turn negatives into positives?

These are the qualities I've seen in the best dancers and learned from the best teachers, and they've served me well in my career and in all aspects of my life. And as I've learned from these amazing teachers and peers, I've discovered something about myself—just as much as I love dancing, I love *teaching* dance. For me, the most rewarding part of my job on *Dancing with the Stars* was teaching my celebrities what to do and watching them blossom.

And what I was teaching them wasn't just the steps to the paso doble or the tango.

I was teaching them about body confidence, about a positive attitude, about dealing with insecurities and fears, about facing the world with your eyes focused and clear. (What you'll read about in part 1.)

I was teaching them about eating in the healthiest way possible, about good nutrition, and about developing a savvy attitude about food. (What you'll read about in part 2.)

I was teaching them about developing a strong core and a powerful, toned body, and improving their overall health. I was helping them find the time to move so that they could recognize what's really important and what all of our bodies, minds, and spirits truly need. (What you'll read about it part 3.)

My celebrity partners and I often talked about why the show is so popular—and the many fans I've met over the years have wanted to discuss this, too. The show isn't just about dancing—it's about transformation. Every viewer who tunes in loves watching the celebrities transform themselves over the course of their journey. They see the initial

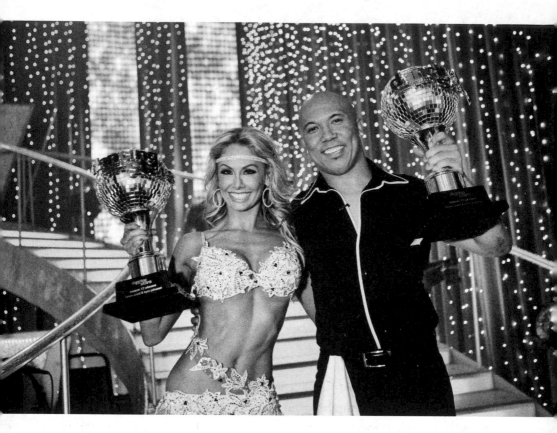

nerves and watch the confidence build slowly. They cheer the contestants as their bodies change, and they take pride in the visible improvements in the dance with each week that passes.

The transformations are utterly believable and thrilling to see because they happen in real time, in front of the viewers' eyes, and they really do work! Good, consistent exercise really works. Good, healthy eating really works. Good doses of confidence really work, too. And both the celebrities and the viewers know that it takes a combination of those three elements to create a Mirror Ball winner.

I've put the best of all of my teaching into this book. I've taught so many different types of people over the years, and this has helped me become more patient and understanding. Trust me, I'm still tough and a stern taskmaster with all of my partners—because you have to be!—but my ultimate goal is always to get the very best out of anyone I'm working with.

It's been incredibly gratifying for me to take someone who is too shy to even look in the mirror that first week of rehearsals and then watch them waltzing on live television for the world to see only weeks later. So I want you to use this book as your very own teacher, and more than anything I want it to enable you to look in the mirror and watch your very own transformation become reality.

Needless to say, I also hope you will have as much fun using this book as I did writing it!

And in case you were wondering where the title came from, well, five, six, seven, and eight were the first numbers I really knew. They represent who I am and what I've known since I was a little girl, and they also prep a dancer's brain for the performance to come.

To me, it means more than dance. It means, "Let's get to it!"

Are you ready?

I know you are . . . it's time to transform how you approach health and wellness. With toning exercises, clean eating, and refreshed confidence.

And a five, six, seven, eight . . . let's get started.

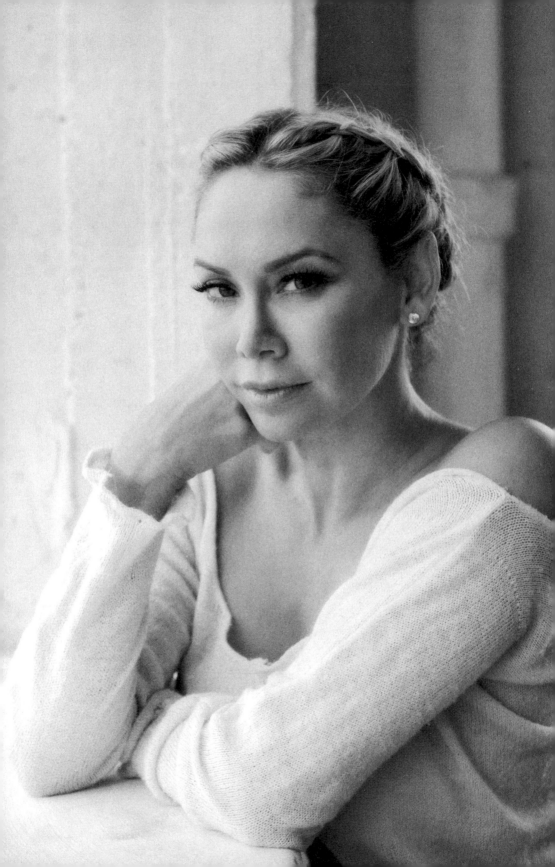

PART I

A DANCER'S LESSONS

With Donny Osmond after winning the season ten championship.

The Ten Commandments of Being a Winner

Few people realize this, but being a winner has very little to do with winning. Life is full of losses and setbacks, and we can't control that—but we can choose how we respond. Win or lose, winners are people who take risks, who aren't afraid to step outside their comfort zones. They set realistic goals and pursue them with a can-do attitude.

I've learned this after many experiences in the dance world. Of course it is always a wonderful feeling to hold that trophy or medal in your hand and have the applause ringing in your ears, but I've been proud of my personal victories along the way as well. I may have lost the competition, but perhaps I developed a wonderful friendship, for example, or learned a new skill, or discovered an unknown talent about myself.

The eating and exercise plans in this book aren't just about toning your muscles—they're about toning your confidence. These ten commandments are the best lessons about confidence I've learned from my dance coaches and many other people who have inspired me over the years. Remember, the first rule of confidence is that it comes from within. No one gets to decide if you're a winner—except you!

1

A Winner Understands the Power of Dreams

I discovered ballroom dancing when I was thirteen—all because my brother had a crush on a girl at school. She took lessons and asked him to join her. I used to go with my mum to pick him up, and I thought that whole world was quite strange because I considered myself to be a "real" dancer doing ballet and jazz and tap. I just thought ballroom dancing was something your grandparents did. Sometimes we'd get there early, though, and I'd watch the dancers and think, *Hmm, this almost looks interesting*.

One day, a boy there didn't have a partner, so the teacher asked me to get up and dance with him. I was instantly in love. No, not with the boy—with the dancing! The music, the accents, the flow, the movement . . . That was the beginning of my ballroom career.

Within a year my professional partner and I were chosen to represent Australia in three different world championships. I felt so privileged to represent my country and saw a huge opportunity in front of me. I made the difficult choice to move to London shortly thereafter to train with some of the world's best teachers. After a few years of study there I competed in one of the world's most prestigious ballroom competitions, the Blackpool Dance Festival, in Blackpool, England. My partner and I placed seventh, which was an incredible triumph for us. We earned an invitation to the Masters in Germany, an invitation-only competition for the best of the best, worldwide. It was incredible and I felt like I'd really arrived as a ballroom dancer.

As strange as it sounds, after we earned our spot at the Masters, I quickly realized that professional ballroom competitions were not for me. I walked away. I knew it was absolutely the right decision because I didn't miss it at all. I only knew I wanted to do something more. Something that was more me.

Around this time, an Australian producer was casting for a show that was going to be like the super-successful *Riverdance*—which showcased Irish step dancing and made it mainstream—only featuring ballroom dancers. It was called *Burn the Floor*, and it's since become an international phenomenon. *What an amazing opportunity*, I thought, because I'd had all that musical theater background but this show was going to be a ballroom musical. I was so incredibly happy when I got cast. I had the opportunity to work with an amazing team and dance alongside some of the world's most talented dancers. My ballroom partner, Tomas, was hired, too, and we performed all over the world, including at Radio City Music Hall in New York City in 1999. I felt like I had finally found where I needed to be—onstage.

This was a truly exciting time for me, and I wanted to have some fun, too! Because I'd spent so much of my youth and adolescent years rehearsing, performing, and traveling I was very driven and focused. But I wanted to let loose. *Burn the Floor* was that opportunity. It was such an exciting time in my life and I got to really get to know myself on my own terms as I performed with the show for six years on and off. Because I listened to my heart, I was finally able to express myself—and become the performer I'd always dreamed of being.

2

Winners Are Willing to Take Risks
and to Get Outside Their Comfort Zones

Over the years, I've gotten used to adapting and stepping out of my comfort zone. Sometimes this was by choice and sometimes this was by necessity. I've worked the front desk in a hotel (and did airport pickups, too). I've been a student, a weather girl, a receptionist, a host, a model, a waitress, a ballroom dancer, a Broadway dancer, a showgirl, a costume decorator, a dance teacher, a dance judge, and, of course, a professional on *Dancing with the Stars*. I've had to learn skills that I can instantly adapt to whatever life throws at me, skills I would have never learned without taking risks.

One of the biggest risks I took—and certainly one of the scariest!—was joining the American cast of *Dancing with the Stars*. After three seasons and a Mirror Ball win in Australia, I felt at home on the show. One of my Australian producers went to America to help them launch the show there, and when he showed them some footage of me, they liked what they saw and asked me to audition for the US show. I was incredibly shocked, but he convinced me to give it a shot and try out. I flew to the US for a series of meetings with the production team, and then went back to Sydney and forgot all about it. A few days later, they called me and told me they needed me there in less than a week! Fortunately, I hadn't yet committed to the Australian show. I knew it would be good for me to have a bit of a change, so I decided to take a leap and make the move.

I was still so shocked at the amazing news that my girlfriends were giddier than I was. They were telling me that I'd really made it big. I was going to Hollywood! Maybe I'd get a famous movie star partner like George Clooney! I laugh at myself now, but on the plane over, I was skimming through *Star* magazine, wondering if my partner would be Leonardo DiCaprio. Can you tell I was slightly delusional? I was just dizzy with nerves and excitement.

I can't begin to put into words what it felt like on my first day of rehearsals, driving my rental car to the famous CBS studios in Hollywood. I grew up watching those wonderful old MGM musicals, and I used to dream that I had been born in that era and could have starred in one of them along with Cyd Charisse or Judy Garland or Gene Kelly. I'd never been to a big studio like that before, ever. I remember thinking, *Oh my gosh, what am I doing here?* Then they waved me over to the parking lot, and my name was there. This nice young woman named Lisl hurried out and said, "Hi, I'm your PA, what can I get you?" My own personal assistant? Me? She showed me to my trailer, and I almost keeled over. I had my own trailer, too! I couldn't believe it. In Australia we do the show in quite a small studio, and the celebrity females and dancers used to share just one trailer.

Talk about shell shock. I had to keep pinching myself to believe that I was living in Hollywood. By the time I got to the rehearsal studio, I didn't know what planet I was on, and I was a bundle of nerves waiting to see which A-lister was going to be my partner.

In walked Jerry Springer.

He looked at me, and he said, "I'm sorry."

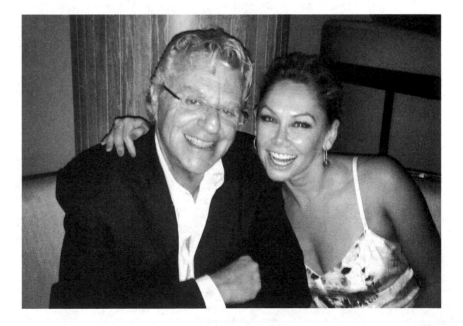

Check Your Ego at the Door

To succeed in something new you have to be open to trying new experiences while conceding that you'll have to step (sometimes leap) outside of your comfort zone. It doesn't hurt to be able to laugh at yourself, too.

I have danced with people who have been so talented and picked up the steps quickly, and I've also had the opposite, where they struggle and find that moving as a couple on a stage, to music, with rhythm, is not natural to them at all. I've gone very far in the competition with people who were not the best dancers, technically speaking, but these competitors embraced the experience and became very endearing to viewers. Everyone saw how hard they tried and how they put their heart and soul into every dance.

No offense intended here, but Jerry Springer is the prime example of that to me. People had a particular view of him because of his talk show, but he wanted to have an incredible experience on the show to honor his daughter and be able to dance with her at her wedding. That resonated in every step he took on the dance floor. Seeing him improve week after week was a journey everyone wanted to share—because it was so easy to relate to and ultimately so very endearing and delightful.

The celebrity dancers I have worked with are the kind of people who are always open to learning, to admitting their flaws—and, more than anything, they quickly learned not to be afraid of looking silly. They were trying their best, and they were doing so with honesty and with a keen sense of fun. I find those skills to be far more valuable than the ability to repeat dance steps quickly.

My best partners had trust and faith in me, the person guiding them. You can translate that to any experience where you may not be the expert. It's important not to criticize yourself when you make a mistake. Be patient with yourself, but never stop wanting to learn. Find a way to be proud of the work you're putting in, and just know that it will come. Sometimes the greatest challenge is following someone else's lead (particularly when you have two left feet!).

I burst out laughing, and so did he.

So he wasn't George Clooney, but he turned out to be the best person I could have had for my first dance partner in America. He was so nice and so smart and kind, with such a beautiful family. We ended up having such a great friendship and remain friends to this day. People loved him on the show—they saw such a different side of him—and he ended up doing really well.

Winners Do What They Love

Working with Donny Osmond on *Dancing with the Stars* was pure joy. Not only did he have a great following, but he was a natural-born performer, overflowing with stage charisma, and, most importantly, he was such a nice person. Read what he has to say in chapter 6, and you'll see what I mean.

The thing with *Dancing with the Stars*—and part of what makes it so compelling to watch—is that you can't really hide who you are. Doing the dances shows the world your true self. And he really, really loved every minute of it. As the weeks went by and I was doing my best to come with routines where he could shine, knowing we were up against tough competition, Donny made me laugh one day when he told me all he really wanted was to do better than his sister, Marie. She'd come in third when she'd been on the show. After we won—and I burst into tears—he immediately looked for Marie in the crowd to rub it in. Even now, he still teases her about it in his Vegas show. Talk about a sibling rivalry! Don't get me wrong; they love each other to bits.

The point is, Donny is one of the hardest-working performers I've ever met, and I have met thousands of driven and determined performers over the years. We were rehearsing for *Dancing with the Stars* all day in Las Vegas, and then he'd drive to the Flamingo and get onstage for a two-hour show where he'd sing and dance and entertain the audience and leave them wanting more. How did he get the energy? I have no idea. He was a machine! What he did was so impressive, but he just loves it. He's got that work ethic and has been doing this since he was a little boy. He's the ultimate professional. Talk about passion! It was impossible not to want to work as he did, and nothing made me happier than seeing his face when we won the Mirror Ball.

On my last season on *Dancing with the Stars*, Robert Herjavec, a highly successful businessman and star of ABC's *Shark Tank*, had such a passion for what we were doing. This passion was so obvious and so genuine, it was infectious—and it was one of the reasons why we advanced as far as we did. I always tell my celebrity partners to walk out onto the floor and believe they are going to be incredible—and to show that confidence to the world. I would often say to Robert, "Let your light shine!"

People want to see that. They want to see you thriving and enjoying what you do. No matter how talented you are as an athlete or a performer, the most important thing is having fun. For instance, one of the competitors on a recent Australian season, Ash Pollard, was known from a celebrity cooking show. She was lovely but communicated her goal from the outset—we all knew she wanted to win the Mirror Ball at all costs.

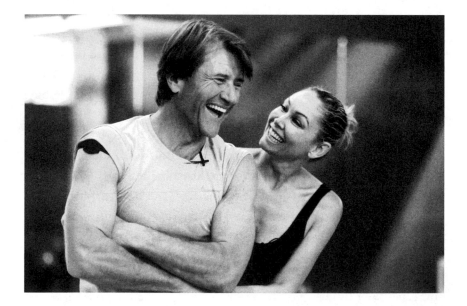

Because she was so aggressively focused on the win, this translated into her dances. They were tough, aggressive, and powerful. Another contestant, Emma Freedman, a well-known TV presenter in Australia, had a bit more fun with it. She was competitive, but the audience related more to her easygoing attitude, and she eventually won the Mirror Ball in September 2015.

What both these contestants learned was that when you want something so badly, it can affect your dancing. Your attitude comes through the dance, and in Ash's case, she wanted it so badly that it made her movement less fluid. The audience didn't respond as well, despite her being an incredible athlete and performer. During the dance, you can think only of the music and the moment, and push the ultimate prize out of your head. The best dancers want only to do their very best in that dance, at that precise instant.

As a viewer and a judge you want to be relaxed and enjoy the performance. When the actress Rumer Willis took part in the tenth-anniversary season of *Dancing with the Stars* in America, she gave her heart and soul to every performance. She was so genuinely passionate about the music and movement during rehearsals and when she was live on that stage, that the viewers could feel it. We were all rooting for her (don't tell Robert though)!

Winners Compete with Themselves
and Are Gracious Even in Defeat

Donny joked about his sibling rivalry with Marie, but I knew that the only person he was actually competing with was himself. My parents taught me early on about the importance of discipline and drive if I wanted to be the best possible dancer, and Donny had the same attitude.

I started going to local dance competitions, called Eisteddfods, when I was about six. My dad made all my props, and we'd pile into the car and off we'd go. I used to win a lot of these competitions and was almost getting a bit too full of myself, almost expecting to win. There was this one particular little girl named Shirley whom I always competed against. I usually beat her, but when she finally won, I was so upset that I burst into tears backstage. Mum came to find me, and there was no sympathy at all. "Stop with those tears and go congratulate Shirley," she told me. I'll never forget her saying that. "What's to cry about?" she went on. "She was better than you today. And if you work hard enough you'll be better than her tomorrow."

So I wiped my eyes, found Shirley, and congratulated her. I realized, even though I was only six, that my mum had just given me an extremely valuable lesson. Because you won't win all the time. The best competition you will ever have is yourself. And this painful loss made me want to work even harder and get even better as a dancer.

You can't be in show business without experiencing rejection. Even the most famous superstars have been rejected at one point or another. We all know that rejections are rarely about us personally. Perhaps the casting director or choreographer needed someone who was a particular physical type. Or who could speak French. Or who looked good with the costars or other partners. Or who could do a very particular dance move that was incredibly difficult (think of Cassie's famous back bend in *A Chorus Line*!).

After so many years of working on *Dancing with the Stars*, all the professional dancers have become very good friends. We all wish each other well and celebrate each other's wins (and empathize over low scores). But at the end of the day, it's still a competition. We all want to come out on top, and even though I really adore everyone, I still want to beat them! That's the whole point. Somebody's going to win—which means everybody else is going to lose.

If my partner and I had done well enough to proceed to the next show, we had to get right to thinking about the next dance. Sometimes, though, someone might have had an off night and was mentally beating themselves up about it (I could instantly tell from their body language if they were upset, and then I'd sit down with them and we would have a nice long chat about it) or maybe they were distressed about their scores.

"Okay, let's forget about that and move on. Let's figure out what we have to do better for the next week," I'd tell them. And if they looked at me skeptically, I'd add, "Honestly, what you just did is forgotten. Let that dance go. We have to start again, from the beginning."

Things Mum Would Say

My mum is the rock of our family and my best friend. She keeps everyone together and is such a positive influence on me. When I was younger, that meant at times instilling a firm sense of discipline, even when I didn't want it. Like all children, there were times when I didn't want to go to class or do all the rehearsing I had to do, and she was the one who kept me on track and pushed me to be the best I could be. She believed in me, supported me, and was firm enough to tell me no and keep my priorities straight when I was too young to see them clearly. Often this advice took the form of her favorite sayings—her dancer's lessons for her dancing daughter:

Practice makes perfect.

If you don't have anything nice to say, don't say anything at all.

Don't make faces; if the wind changes it will stay that way. (I think in America, your version is, "You face will freeze that way!")

If at first you don't succeed, try and try again.

No use crying over spilled milk.

If you're too sick to go to school, you're too sick to hold your head up high.

Honesty's the best policy.

More haste, less speed.

You'll thank me for this one day.

If you count your pennies the pounds will take care of themselves.

Be a good listener.

The early bird catches the worm.

Jealousy's a curse.

Look before you leap.

Be nice to each other. (That was usually followed by: "I don't care who started it!")

I'd tell them the exact same thing when they were on a high from getting their best score ever, too.

Sometimes a no is as good as a yes. You can't look at it as losing. You need to realize that hearing no is just another experience and an opportunity to try something new. Use any upset or frustration as fuel to motivate you to get out there and do it again. I've been to countless auditions and been told I wasn't the right fit. When that happened, I was disappointed, but I also knew that I wasn't going to lose any sleep over decisions that were out of my control. When I was eliminated early in the competition with David Hasselhoff, I struggled because we wanted to perform and have fun—but we had clearly been told no by the voters and unfortunately had an early exit that season. My next partner was Hines Ward, and I took a

Push the Jealousy Away . . .
Because Everyone Has a Different Skill Set

During my early dance training, I was always doing group performances with the other kids in my class. We all knew, even at such an early age, who was good at splits and who was the best tumbler and who had the most beautiful extension. There was no point in being jealous. Everyone's body was different and everyone's skills were different. Our teachers encouraged us to work harder on our specific skills and talents, and to admire and appreciate the talents of everyone else without envy. I learned if I liked someone's costume better or if she had better turns or was more flexible, I had to work harder to beat that person. I had to own my own costume. I had to be proactive on my own turns. Not consume myself with envy.

But it wasn't always easy. I would go to state championships, and if I won, I'd hear things like, "What were the judges thinking? I don't know if she deserved to win. Do you?" being said by people who wanted me to hear it. My mum was very good at helping me let it go in one ear and out the other.

"You can't take that on board," she'd say. "You are better than that."

totally different approach with him. We looked at each week as a win. We were motivated by the small victories. We literally took it step by step instead of saying "We know we are going to win the whole thing" from day one. Because we focused only on the present—not on the long-term goal of winning the competition—the small, incremental wins allowed us to recognize how well we were working together and how much better we could be.

The takeaway from this, of course, is that just because something happened this week doesn't mean it's going to happen next week. You'll always have another opportunity. It may be a different opportunity, but it will be a real one just the same.

What this really means: you have to lose to know how it feels to really win.

In the dance world, I'm sorry to say, jealousy is a big thing, along with backstabbing and spite. Other dancers might say mean things to try to put you off your game or psych you out. Sometimes they'll elbow you out of the way, trying to cut you out so you can't get to your space on the floor.

Pathetic, isn't it? But some people just have to win. I knew enough to know that when that happened it wasn't about trying sabotage me personally. The competition was so important to them that they had to come out on top.

I'm so thankful I was never like that. I've learned how to be tough and strong, but I will always know that I've gotten where I have by being kind, not mean. I haven't been that ruthless person, stepping over someone to get where I am. I've always won whenever I ran my own race—and, as you know, competed with myself first. That has always kept me grounded. And motivated!

Of course, it's human nature to be envious at times. Instead of focusing on the jealousy, flip it right on its head and do what I did. Spur yourself on to be the best at what you and only you can do. At the end of the day, that's all that really matters.

A Winner Is Present and in the Moment

Doesn't it make you crazy when you see someone driving on the highway, drinking a coffee and talking on their cell phone? Multitasking can be useful when you truly have a million things to get done (and find a way to do it safely!), but it's a killer for dancers. You have to be so present and in the moment when you're performing, or you will flop. You'll never get the best out of yourself otherwise.

When I know I'm in it, truly absorbed into that moment on that floor, that's when it seems like I could practically fly to the moon and back, it feels so good. It means I'm fully focused and all my senses are engaged in doing each step and turn and dip the way it's meant to be done. In that moment, I'm totally engaged in the dance. It's all flowing. I'm in the zone.

My partners on the show quickly learned as the weeks went on that if they were thinking about the next step and worrying that they would mess it up, they almost certainly would mess it up. One of the hardest things for them to learn was how to concentrate solely on what we were doing that day. They were often way too hard on themselves, saying that they should have done this step or they shouldn't have missed that one . . . or wondering and being apprehensive about what they might have to do next week. My job was to bring them back to the moment and to clear their heads of anything but what we were doing in rehearsals. Easier said than done! That's why we rehearsed as much as possible—it allowed the actual steps to become second nature, and all the focus could shift to actually performing them, in the moment.

Being present and in the moment is a powerful tool for all aspects of life. It helped me in auditions, and it will help you in meetings or situations where you need to focus solely on the task at hand. If you're well prepared and have training to fall back on, whatever your profession, your instincts will kick in and you'll know what to do. Try your utmost to concentrate on the now. You can't endlessly worry about what happened in the past, because it's done; and you can't predict the future, because it hasn't happened yet. Get out there on your own stage of the moment and show the world what you can do!

6

A Winner Has a Can-Do Attitude—

Don't Say You Can't Do It, Because You Can Do It!

How can I tell if someone's not a confident dancer? I can see it instantly, in their eyes. When I have the chance to judge on the show, I know that if the celebrity's eyes are wandering, it means they don't know what they're doing. They might be smiling, but they don't give off a confident vibe. I always told my partners to fix their eyes in the direction we were meant to be going. It makes them look confident and at ease, even if their nerves are churning inside!

After all, how many times did your parents tell you to look where you were going? That advice isn't just about not tripping on an uneven sidewalk—it's about confidence. If you walk into a job interview with your eyes fixed on the personnel director, extend your hand, smile warmly, and greet the person politely and firmly, you will have already made a stunning impression. Look hesitant or nervous, and you'll never get hired, even if you're the most qualified candidate on paper.

As soon as you doubt yourself it's over. You can't second-guess yourself. I've done that before and things have gone wrong. If I doubt myself onstage, the audience knows. If I doubt myself when walking into an interview or an audition, I'll never get the job.

One way I motivate myself is with music. It always puts me in a good place, and it's always the cue—probably because of years of dance training—for my body to get going! After a long day of rehearsals I would be exhausted from teaching but know I had to do something for myself. I'd be at home thinking that I should really head to that Pilates class or get out and go for that walk. I'd turn up my favorite songs, blare the speakers, and let the music take over to get me moving again. I had to really push myself, but I'm not a quitter—and the music always helped me find the energy I needed. I knew that once I was there at the class or out on the walk, it would make me feel so much better. And if I was very tired and the class was very hard, I'd listen to my body and scale it back a little bit—but still be proud of myself with the quiet satisfaction of having done the work I knew was good for me.

Often, with my celebrities, I would use the Mental Countdown technique. This can be very useful for you, too. Especially when, for example, you know you really want to do your exercises but you're having a really bad day. The kids are screaming, you burned the dinner, and you want to just crawl into a cool, quiet, dark hole and cry. That's when the excuses can start, and it's totally understandable. Believe me, I heard so many excuses from my partners, but it was my job to say, "Okay, I hear you, but, no, we can do this." I would make a deal with them. "Let's do it five more times, then you can take a break or eat something."

That always worked. We would do the dance five more times, or the exercises five more times, and I would count them down. Many exercise teachers do this during their classes, telling their students. "Okay, we're going to do this for thirty seconds." They do something very difficult for that time, and when the teacher has reached 5-4-3-2-1, they say, "Great job. Let's do it for another fifteen!" The students will already be doing it and in the zone, and they keep at it. It works every time.

Other times, dancers are in a situation where we haven't had time to rehearse the routine. At auditions, we quickly learn a new piece of choreography and we know we have to get it right or we'll not be asked on to the next round. Frankly, sometimes we have to fake it until we make it. You've really just got to put your best self out onto the floor, show your personality, and get as many of the steps out as you possibly can in the short amount of time you're given. That's better than trying to get everything right and not focusing on connecting with the audience or casting director.

I remember days when I was performing in *Burn the Floor* on Broadway and I would wake up feeling too exhausted to get out of bed. We had eight shows a week as well as rehearsals, and the energy we needed to wow everyone was intense. But the show must go on, and it had to go on with me in it! I had to psych myself up and just mentally put myself in the position of, "I'm going to do this." There's a famous phrase that every showgirl hears as soon as she's been in a show for a while: "T and T, darling. It's a tits and teeth night!"

What this means is, sometimes it's hard to psych yourself up to bring your all when you're doing the same show night after night, week after week. Anyone who works at a job where you're basically doing the same tasks for a large part of your workday knows exactly what this is about!

On a T & T night, I just didn't feel good or was so exhausted that I didn't know how I was going to perform at my best. My fellow dancers and stagehands always knew when that was happening to me or anyone else—everyone went through it!—and they'd laugh and tease us about its being a T & T night.

But then the lights would go down and the curtain would go up, and I would be on the stage and the adrenaline would kick in. Somehow, I'd summon the energy and do my very best. I'd psych myself up by dancing a little bit differently or trying to catch someone else's eye and give them an extra-big smile. They'd smile back, so happily. And I knew I'd make it through the rest of the performance.

I always got through my T & T nights thanks to something I'd seemingly heard a million times from my first dance teacher, Miss Bernie: "Don't you dare come off the stage halfway through a routine if you forget your steps," she used to say to us all the time. "Just keep doing it!"

In other words, fake it till you make it! Who will know the difference? Only you will!

If I didn't have the time to properly rehearse, and then it was suddenly time to perform and give the audience the razzle-dazzle they were expecting, then it was time to fake it until I made it and let my showmanship and professionalism do the job.

Years later, I often thought of Miss Bernie when I was choreographing on *Dancing with the Stars*, because I was able to bring a bit of theatricality into my routines and tell my partners, "Don't worry if you forget your steps. Just keep doing it!"

Robert Herjavec was a perfect example of this. He was the first to admit he was an inexperienced dancer before the show, but he sure knew how to fake it.

"In any environment," he told me many times during our rehearsals, "the ability to sell yourself better than your competitor is often what gets you a deal, or what leaves you walking away empty-handed." And his wonderful confidence and pleasure in dancing weren't faked at all.

Being Confident Is Not Being Pushy!

We see this all too often, and I'm constantly debating this with my girlfriends. Women can be perceived differently than men when it comes to being confident. A man who knows his mind is often described as forceful or strong or in command; a woman who does the same is often insulted and called pushy. That drives me crazy!

All the female professionals on *Dancing with the Stars* were the "bosses" of our partners. We knew what had to be done and we had to communicate that effectively. We were working with men at the top of their game in their respective professions, and they were often not used to being completely at the mercy of a woman telling them what to do. That sometimes compounded their vulnerability and insecurities, because whatever they were good at in their successful careers didn't much matter in a dance studio (well, the athletes and performers did have the physical strength and grace, but none of them were professional dancers).

Sometimes, these celebrities may have thought they were doing better than they actually were, and they didn't want to listen. It was very challenging for me not to be intimidated, especially since, like many performers (believe it or not!), I am actually quite a shy person. But at the end of the day I knew I was a good teacher and could do a good job. I believed in myself and my training and my skills as a teacher. That was the big difference that allowed me to put my foot down in the beginning when I knew I had to—otherwise we would have failed as partners. I had to remain strong and say, "You know what? I'm the boss on the dance floor, so you're going to have to listen to what I say, and listen to it now."

And you know what? That was always the turning point in so many of my partnerships. I earned the respect of my partners by laying down the rules and telling them how to work and succeed in my environment. They relaxed, because they knew they were in safe hands and I would do my very best to see them excel on the dance floor.

This also made it much easier for me to stick up for myself in other situations, too. When I was on *The Celebrity Apprentice*, I was in a boardroom—which was about as different from the casual freedom of a dance studio as possible—and was soon being thrown under the bus by colleagues in a challenging situation. But I knew what I was getting into, and I was very proud of myself for signing on in the first place. I not only got out of my comfort zone, but I saw how effective a woman's confidence can be in a business setting. Think of this next time you are faced with challenges at work. "No" is a powerful word. Demanding respect is often the only way you can hope to get it, too.

7

A Winner Sets Realistic Goals

One of the reasons the Mental Countdown technique is so effective is that it breaks down your perception of the exercise and how long it takes into small increments.

I'll discuss this more in chapter 6, but I've found that the dancer's habit of breaking down every single step helps me with all the tasks I need to do. That's why when I am starting to choreograph a dance, I get out my notepad and write down a whole line of eights, for the count of the music, which allows me to break the dance down into a beginning, a middle, and an end. There is a system to it, and writing it down makes my job so much easier.

Think about this when you're starting to change the way you eat and train. Start small. If you walked into a gym for the very first time and saw all the machines there, of course you'd be overwhelmed—unless you had someone show you the ropes and break it all down for you. Then you'd realize it's actually quite simple and certainly not intimidating.

I've also found that a to-do checklist is a useful tool, not only for keeping track of all the things I have to do and places I have to be, but because it is extremely satisfying when you finish some of your tasks and can cross them off the list. Even if what you need to do is no more complicated than going to the post office or taking the kids to the park, knowing you finished what you set out to do keeps you going! So keep a small notepad and pen in your handbag, or use an app on your smartphone.

Another way to break it down is to state your goal or goals. Say them aloud. Write them down. Acknowledge them. Most of all, be realistic about them.

Let's say you know you want to lose thirty pounds. That's a lot, and it's an extremely admirable goal. What I would do is say, "I want to lose thirty pounds, but my goal for now is to lose ten." That is a much more attainable goal and will come to you more quickly.

Then, when you've lost ten pounds, you can say, "I wanted to lose thirty pounds, and I am so proud of myself for already losing ten. Way to go! Now I am going to lose another ten. When I do, I will then only have ten more pounds to go."

Doing this will not only make your goal less scary but will reinforce how hard you are working toward it. For example, *Dancing with the Stars* had, ultimately, fourteen dances over ten weeks. The ultimate goal was to win the Mirror Ball, but the more realistic goal was to get through every week with a high enough score so we could advance. Every week was different, and we could, as you know by now, only focus on that one dance. That goal was attainable.

Part of starting and working toward your goals is getting prepared. Doing your homework will give you the knowledge you need to smooth the path. You might realize that what you thought you wanted isn't something you actually want at all, and you'll chuck those plans and move on to something else. But the only way to fine-tune your needs is to learn everything you can about what you're hoping and planning to do.

And then even when you know you're doing your job well and have mastered the skills needed to keep on doing so, you still need to do your homework. On every season of the show, I would set realistic goals. Of course I wanted to win the Mirror Ball, but you can't be thinking about the finale when there are still weeks and weeks to go. You have to focus on the present and be there in the moment. (All the skills you just read about!) And then, all of a sudden, hopefully you realize, Wow, I'm in the semifinal—how did that happen?

Well, it happened in large part because I coached my partner to do his very best, and because I always did my homework. I had to be prepared, every literal step of the way. After rehearsals, I would go home and plan ahead. I'd think about the moves, the song to request, the costumes. I'd work out the entire routine so it was fresh in my head and I didn't have to spend any rehearsal time changing it. This allowed me so much more time to actually do what I did best—teach and dance!

When I first met Robert Herjavec, he surprised me when he told me how much he knew about the show before he even got cast. He also told me that having done his homework made the experience more fun and gave him a competitive advantage over the other celebrities. *Dancing with the Stars* had been one of his mother's favorite shows, he explained. When she became quite ill with cancer, he used to go to the hospital and watch the show with her and the other women in the oncology ward. It made her happy to see it, and it made him happy to be with her. Robert never thought in a million years that he would be asked to do the show, but his mom always told him that that's how he would know he was a big star who had finally "arrived." So when he was asked to be on the show, he didn't even question it. He was ready! Tragically, Robert's mother passed away before he was cast, but in some ways it made it even more special for him to be a part of it.

When you're doing the homework for the exercise section of this book, the very first assignment is to see your physician, if you haven't had a recent checkup, and get the go-ahead for a new fitness regimen. (This is crucial for everyone, but especially for those who may have underlying health issues.) Then, think through your fitness goals. Start small, as you know already. I know you can do it!

8

A Winner Expects the Unexpected—
and Knows How to Pivot

I work in a business where every day is different. Every rehearsal is different, every performance is different, and every audience is different. It's helped me learn to expect the unexpected. Of course you don't want anything negative to be the unexpected—like *Burn the Floor* losing its financing—but when you are prepared and have a contingency plan, it's easier to deal with any surprising situation.

Actually, I can't believe that I'm the age I am and still dancing. I never thought in a million years that I'd be doing this. I'm so grateful for it. But you're always wondering, *When is this going to end?* When I had my injury with Hines Ward back in 2011, it changed my perspective. I remember lying there in that hospital and thinking, Oh my gosh, this could be it, what else am I going to do? And feeling so lucky that I didn't have to make that decision then.

Sometimes I get nervous and scared about my future like everybody does, but now I'm excited. I don't know if it's what I've learned from dancing and being so disciplined, but I'm just ready for the next chapter and putting things in place. I think for a dancer or professional athlete the worst thing is to think that you're going to do this forever and ever. It's a fine line though, because you do want to be in the moment and present and put all of your energies into that—which is the best you can be at dancing.

What this means is, I've always known that sometimes you need to pivot in your career. As a dancer I'm constantly reinventing myself, learning new skills, and pivoting during a dance when the choreography calls for it. You never know when you're going to get the next job or get injured. That makes show business exciting but it's also very scary. You have to get up and get out there and bring it every time. You also have to be okay rolling with the punches. And be prepared to pivot on a dime. That's life, isn't it?

It's always going to be unpredictable. Like I said, head up, eyes forward, focus on where you're going, and go for it!

One of the earliest times that I remember making a shift in my career and pivoting was after I took a break from training in London. I returned home to Australia and my mum encouraged me to try something new. I was also in desperate need of some pocket money, so it was time to get a job outside of dance. I went to a hospitality college and ended up getting a job at the front desk of the International Motor Hotel. I loved it! When you work in a service job, not only do you see so many personalities, but you have to stand there with a smile and instantly anticipate their needs. (Which, not surprisingly, really helped me years later on *Dancing with the Stars*, when I worked with celebrities who were very nervous. Being able to read their body language helped us all!) I was a bit cheeky and used to up-sell the rooms—when new guests arrived I'd say we only had a deluxe room available. The owners loved me for that and started me on the night shift because I'd always sell the whole hotel. I found it quite a fun challenge—maybe that was just me being competitive!—to get every room sold. The owners even taught me how to drive the minivan with a stubborn stick shift for the airport pickups. I'd be dressed in my nice uniform for the reception desk, and then the owner would take care of the lobby and I'd drive over to the airport, pick up the guests, drive back, run behind the desk, and check the guests in.

At the same time, I continued to take ballroom dancing lessons and teach children as well. The hotel owners loved my dancing—they were like family at this point—so they more or less sponsored me to get back into the competitive world. I got a new partner from Lithuania, Tomas Atkocevicius, who was a beautiful dancer, and we went back to England to train. I got a job at a Holiday Inn in London, putting on an English accent because nobody could understand my Aussie drawl! And because Tomas wasn't able to get working papers, he and I both worked as assistants decorating dance costumes on the side for extra cash to pay for our super-expensive dance lessons. Sometimes we'd literally be up all night sewing. It was intense. Now I can look back on this experience fondly and realize all that hard work was worth it. I had to make a change to reflect on my career thus far and take account of what I'd accomplished. Had I not been open to pivoting—to returning to Australia and getting a job at the hotel—I may not have had the same appreciation and love for dance. It renewed my focus and made me even hungrier to succeed.

Sometimes all you need to do is step back from your current situation and make a bit of a change to see a large impact. Think about that for a second—when's the last time you tried something new? Or pivoted entirely? This could be something as large as a career choice or as small as trying a new yoga class. Change is good and can give you the perspective you need. Just keep an open mind to pivoting—because the strongest lesson you can take away here is how to be adaptable to whatever life throws your way.

9

A Winner Admits When Something's Not Working and Walks Away . . . Even When It's Really Hard

I've always had good instincts about when to make important life transitions. That could be because of my dancer personality. I know my career won't last forever and I can feel the wear and tear on my body more than ever. Pivoting is a dancer's concept at its origin, but it applies so well in this situation.

As a young dancer, I was used to just being solo in the competitions but was thrilled when I discovered my love for ballroom dancing. When I was fourteen I got my first real partner, a sweet boy named Jason. We made it to the finals of the Australian championships, which was pretty big for two beginners! And then I got asked by Grant, the Australian champion at the time, to be his partner. I was so excited! Until I realized how badly this would hurt Jason. I told my mum I was going to call him to let him know and she said, "Oh no, you won't," and drove me to his house. I walked in and was stunned to see a little shrine set up in a corner of the living room with photos of us dancing together. My heart sank. I sat down and told Jason and he was devastated and I felt absolutely terrible.

But I knew the only way I would ever get better was with a partner much more skilled than I was. Grant and I soon became the talk of the Australian ballroom world as I was so young and still a ballroom beginner, really, and because I had come from the ballet and jazz world. (I was still only fourteen and he was seventeen.) We ended up representing Australia in three different world championships, as only one of two couples from each country. It all happened very quickly. I was still doing my other dance training until I was sixteen. I remember my last ballet exam, at the intermediate level, being just too difficult. Not only did I know that I was never going to be a ballerina—I didn't have the right body type and I was always more of a musical theater or showgirl—but my heart wasn't in the ballet world anymore.

So I threw myself into the super-competitive world of professional ballroom dancing and quickly realized that the cost factor greatly added to the mix. It's not like there was big prize money, and the lessons and the travel and the costumes were extremely expensive. I was so lucky and so grateful that my mum paid for all my costumes—I know they cost a fortune. Fortunately, we got a sponsor who helped us when we were representing Australia, along with a stipend to train in London when I was eighteen. We needed to be based there as it was where all the best teachers were and offered quick access to all the competitions in Europe. I was thrilled because I was really adventurous and very driven to be the best.

But when Grant and I split up, I had no regrets about going back to Australia. It was time.

And then, a few years later, Tomas and I were doing very well in the European championships. We placed seventh in Blackpool, which was a huge step forward for us, and were then asked to an invitation-only competition in Germany.

Each couple had to dance two rounds, and we were all on the floor together. As I was concentrating on our tango with my lovely partner, I had a sudden flash: What am I doing, dancing around with all of these other couples? I want to perform. I spend so much time working at all these jobs just to pay for my costumes and shoes and our airplane tickets, and this is not the future I want to have anymore. I want to do so much more. I love this, but I don't see where it's going anymore.

The music stopped and we came off the floor, and I said, "Tomas, look, I love this, it's been incredible, but I don't want to do it anymore."

He stared at me in shock. "How can you say this to me in the middle of a competition?" he asked, appalled.

"Don't worry!" I said quickly. "I'm going to dance this competition and be the best I can be, but this is it . . ."

We went back out and did our best, and placed outside of the top three.

It was the last ballroom competition I ever did.

And I have no regrets about it whatsoever!

Funnily enough, many years later, I knew it was time to leave *Burn the Floor* when I was cast on *Dancing with the Stars*. It was a difficult decision to leave because the show was such a big part of my life and I'd been with the production from the very beginning. But I knew *Dancing with the Stars* presented an exciting and different opportunity. I had to take a risk, pivot, and recognize that this chance was too good to pass up. I parted with the producers amicably, and years later they asked me back when the show came to Broadway in 2009.

Even if you anticipate that feelings might be hurt and someone else's workload increased, when it's time to move on, you need to make the right decision for you. I am a shy person and basically such a people-pleaser that I could have let my sympathies for other people's feelings overrule my better judgment about my own needs. Thank goodness I listened to my instincts. And if you don't stand up for what is right for you, who will? Listen to your heart, and then speak up. This is not being selfish. This is being your own person and having the right to a healthy, happy, and fulfilling life.

10

A Winner Embraces Life

After the thrilling moment of winning the Mirror Ball with Donny Osmond, we flew straightaway to New York to tape *Good Morning America* and talk to the press. I knew I would be spending the next three months there as I'd been asked to appear in *Burn the Floor* on Broadway, with Maksim Chmerkovskiy.

I only had two days of rehearsals before we opened on Thanksgiving. It was such an exciting time. I rented a beautiful apartment with floor-to-ceiling windows overlooking Times Square, and as I'd stare down at all the people hurrying this way and that, and all the cars and buses and taxis speeding by, it was overwhelmingly wonderful. Especially for an Australian. The real New York! A Broadway show! I'd really made it, I told myself. In fact, that was one of those moments where I felt like I had everything I'd ever wanted to have.

But . . . I wasn't fulfilled or happy because I didn't have anyone to share it with. I'd leave the theater at the stage door, with loads of people waiting to see me, the fans who loved *Dancing with the Stars*, taking photos and asking me to sign autographs. They were all so happy and this filled me with joy. But then I'd walk back to my beautiful apartment and be all alone. My boyfriend at the time was in England and things weren't going great with us. I was really feeling sorry for myself.

It's funny how now everything makes sense. You know, with people, it's like you wish for this and you wish for that and then you get it—and you sit back and realize it's not what you expected. I wasn't happy. I'd lost my emotional balance. I was guilty at the time of looking at what I didn't have instead of appreciating the amazing success of winning with Donny and starring on Broadway. I wish I had been more grateful back then instead of wallowing in self-pity. I was focusing on that negative and not enjoying the process of being in New York. I could have gone out and made new friends, but I was exhausted and feeling sorry for myself. And

I doubt that anyone asking for my autograph could have imagined just how sad and lonely I really was at the time!

It wasn't like me not to focus on the positive, and my wonderful mum came to spend Christmas with me after my boyfriend told me he couldn't make it. I also got my divine little dog, Lola, and that helped, too. She was such a Broadway baby and spent every evening in my dressing room when I went onstage!

When the show ended, I went back to Los Angeles and ended things with my boyfriend. I gave him an ultimatum, telling him I wanted to move in together and maybe think about getting married and having kids. I knew, deep down, that this would scare him off—I could have kept the relationship going, but it wouldn't have truly gone anywhere. Donny Osmond, who has a long and loving marriage, was the one who sparked me to do this, because he kept telling me that I needed to *know*. I had to be able to make plans for my future.

Needless to say, I was very upset about being on my own again. Well, I told myself, at least I've still got my job.

And then the phone rang. I didn't have a job, after all. The producers told me that even though I'd just won, they couldn't find a partner suitable for me for the upcoming season of *Dancing with the Stars*. I don't know if they wanted to try some new people out, which was totally understandable, or if they knew my heart was broken and they wanted to give me a break. It didn't really matter. I was humiliated. Devastated. Shocked. After seven seasons, I was off the show.

I really had to pivot and figure out my next move—and in a hurry. What was I going to do? I found myself really lonely in Los Angeles and told myself that, okay, I'd had a really good run of it, but I should probably move back to Australia and meet some nice Aussie boy and try to figure things out. So I did what I always did when I was really upset and called my mum, crying. I told her I had no boyfriend and no job and I was so sad and life was just awful.

"Well," she said after patiently listening to me sob my heart out, "you've worked really hard to get to where you have in the States. You know you have. And a lot of girls would kill to be in your position. I think you should try to stay there. See what else you can do. Give it a go for a while. Think about it."

Eventually, I dried my eyes and started thinking about it. My competitive, positive nature came flooding back. Enough sadness and negativity. *What can I do?* I wondered. *How can I turn this nightmare into some kind of positive?*

That's when I got creative. And proactive with my pivot into my future. I approached *E! News* and pitched myself as a correspondent for the show. I had absolutely nothing to lose—and they went for it! They had me on for the whole season as their *Dancing with the Stars* correspondent, which turned out to be a fantastic move. I was doing something different and learning a new skill set. At first, I have to admit, I was a bit embarrassed to walk onto set and to see all of my friends who were still on the show, but I quickly got over it. I was having a lot of fun, and it was a terrific new challenge. I was talking about something that I obviously knew about, and my producer helped me with the interview questions. Everyone was relaxed and happy to talk to me because they knew me, so that made it a lot easier, too.

And then, much to my surprise, a *Dancing with the Stars* producer came up to me and told me how sorry they were I wasn't on anymore, and how much they missed me—and they asked me to come back. What a wonderful day that was! I was partnered with David Hasselhoff and we were eliminated after the first episode, but that allowed me to go straight back to corresponding for *E!* again and be on the show. I was in heaven. I had the best of both worlds! It all worked out in the end.

At my lowest point, when my job and my relationship were crumbling around me, I was so lucky to have my mum be there for me. Everyone needs someone who believes in them, who pushes them and can see the forest for the trees. My mum was that person at that time. Without her wisdom and encouragement, I might have packed up my bags and fled home to Australia, and I doubt I would have been asked back on the show. It would have been much easier for me to run away from my problems, but I'm glad that I walked into that studio and faced those fears and stuck it out.

And what enabled me to make that pivot was thinking outside the

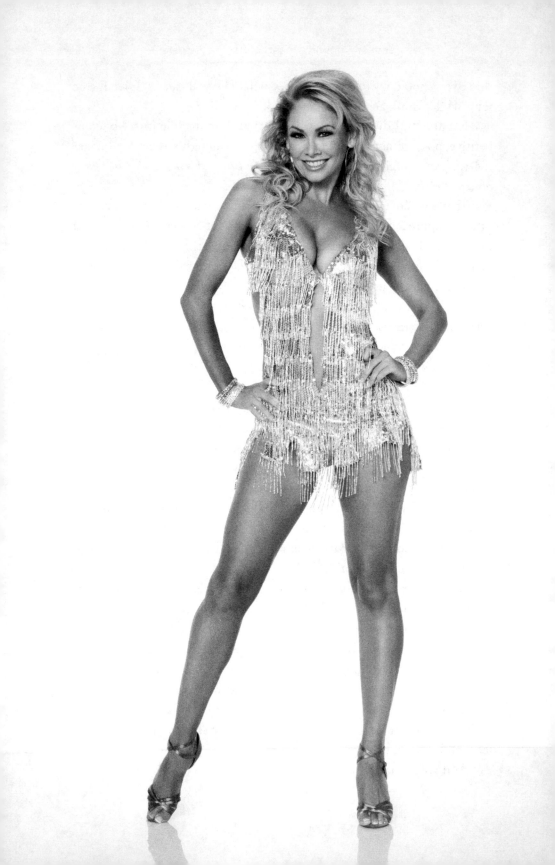

box. I had to ask myself some tough questions, and I had to throw myself out there and try to do something untested. I had to fall back on all the lessons in this chapter to do so—and now I'm happier than I've ever been.

●●●●

What I learned most of all is that embracing life, even at your lowest point, is something you really can't fake. When you do embrace it, you'll get the best out of it. Even when you find yourself in the most painful of situations, embrace it. Own it. It's not going to own you—you're going to own it!

In my last season on the show, Robert Herjavec helped me embrace something I could have been taking for granted. He made me appreciate what I do, because he was the most enthusiastic celebrity I have ever worked with. He just genuinely had such a love and passion for dance. It wasn't just that it reminded him of his beloved mother, but he was in heaven on the dance floor!

"This is so beautiful," he said to me during our first week of rehearsals. "I can't believe you're teaching me how to dance. This is incredible! I'm actually doing a waltz! I'm actually dancing!"

Which brings me back full circle to the first item on my list in this chapter. Put your dreams into action. The biggest gains can come from the biggest risks. The worst that can happen is you get rejected. And then you will regroup, pivot, and figure out a better way to move forward. Live with passion. Find your purpose. And be the healthiest and strongest person you can be. Read on—and I'll show you how!

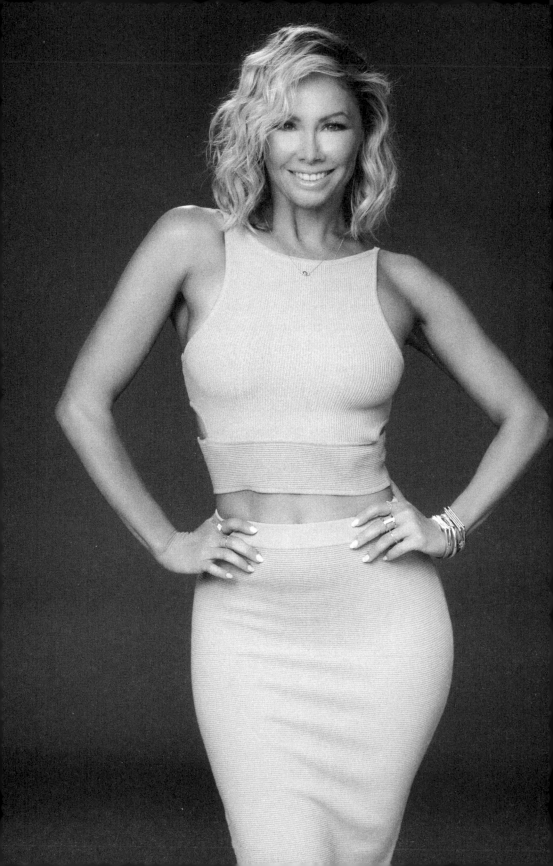

PART II

THE 5-6-7-8
DIET PLAN

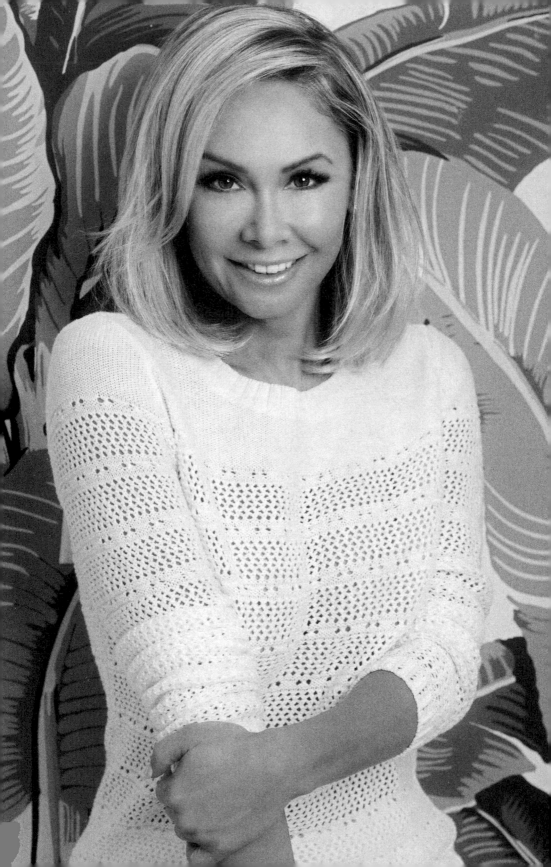

②

My Diet Philosophy

I have been lucky enough to travel the world with dance—to experience and explore different cultures, sights, smells, sounds, and, oh yes, foods!

I'm the kind of person that likes to live life to the fullest. I don't like to feel that I'm depriving myself and missing out, and I particularly love being social and trying new things. I want to be happy, not hungry!

So I've devised a healthy diet philosophy, based on my need as a dancer to eat a super-nutritious diet that gives my body the fuel it requires for maximum performance (don't I sound like a car?!). I've gotten great advice from other dancers, choreographers, teachers, and nutritionists over the years, too. We all have the same goal: to eat well, and to take pleasure in our food. Follow these tips, and you'll be doing the same.

First Off, Dancers Do Eat!

All dancers are in tune with their bodies because they use them for their work. We eat! We have to. For us, food is fuel, and it's as important to us as the shoes we wear and the core exercises we do in the gym.

When I was much younger, I would sometimes see dancers who seemed to survive on nothing more than endless cups of coffee and cigarettes. They might have gotten away with it for a short time because they were so young, but believe me, every professional dancer I've ever worked with has a sound diet plan. If we don't eat well, we don't have energy—and it will show. We are not going to put our careers at risk by following fad diets or starving ourselves!

Luckily, I love vegetables and fruits. I eat a very clean diet, with food prepared simply and well. I like seasoning and strong flavors. I've gotten to a place where I don't crave sugary treats. I don't eat "fake" foods. And if I'm going to indulge in something I don't normally eat—like pizza or pasta—then I am going to savor every morsel. And work out extra-hard the next day!

Clear Out Your Kitchen

Now that you're thinking about changing the way you eat, it's also time to get ruthless and clear out those shelves in your kitchen. And you know why? Because if it isn't there, you can't eat it!

I've worked with a company called Freshology before, and they were great because they would provide well-balanced meals and snacks; the food was healthy and delicious and it took all the guesswork out of what to eat at mealtimes. This also meant that any temptations were minimized. At the studio where we taped *Dancing with the Stars*, we also had an area where we could make fresh juices and smoothies, and we all loved to take advantage of that.

You'll be given lots of ideas about what to eat in the next chapters, but before you start, have a good look at what you tend to prepare for meals. Are there a lot of packaged foods? Is your freezer full of microwaveable meals? Are your pots and pans gathering dust? Time for a deep kitchen cleanse.

You might want to ask a friend over to help you toss the preservative-and-sodium-drenched, fat-and-sugar-laden packaged foods you won't be eating anymore. Have a clear-out party and have fun while you empty the shelves. Keep the staples, like whole grains, flour (switch to whole-wheat or other grains), rice (switch to brown), dried beans and legumes, canned and frozen veggies (especially tomatoes, for making sauce), healthy soups and sauces, and nuts. Get rid of everything else.

And if you hate wasting food as much as I do, try to donate your unwanted items to your local food bank or shelter.

Eat All Day—Especially Healthy Snacks!

A lot of celebrities who appeared on *Dancing with the Stars* asked the professional dancers about how they eat. They watched us, and then they emulated us, because they wanted to be as healthy as we are. They saw us eating a lot more protein and a lot more salads than they often ate—and more than anything else, they saw us eating all the time!

Nearly every dancer I know eats often, all day, every day. We just eat small portions when we do. The reason? It's very hard to dance on a stomach full of a regular-sized or, especially, a dinner-sized meal. It just takes too long to digest, and the energy our bodies need for digestion then gets diverted away from our muscles. The solution is constant snacking on health foods that are easy to digest. As a dancer, you actually eat more frequently throughout the day—but you eat less overall! In addition, snacking on the right kinds of foods keeps your metabolism up and your blood sugar steady, so your cravings for junk food and sugar will lessen.

I also tend to eat early in the day. I love a big breakfast and have whole-grain toast in the morning. I try to minimize the carbs I eat, but when I have them I do it in the morning so I can burn them off throughout the day.

If it's hard for you to eat this way at work, and I know it can be for a lot of people, then try to eat the biggest meal as early in the day as possible. That means a big breakfast, or a big lunch if you're not a breakfast person. And see if you can keep healthy snacks like almonds or grapes at your desk, which will make it much less tempting to go to the snack room.

Or try this. On weekends or days when you're not at work, have a high tea—only make it healthy. A regular high tea is a lovely English tradition where an assortment of sandwiches, savory bites, and lots of little desserts are brought out one by one, along with endless cups of tea . . . and cream and sugar! Just hold the cream and sugar! It's not exactly a low-calorie meal, but it's so much leisurely fun, and I can never eat much more for the rest of the day after enjoying one. I'll show you how to have your own 5-6-7-8 version of a high tea on page 282 in chapter 11. It's a terrific way to move your dinnertime so you won't be eating a large, heavy meal at night.

I've also gotten into the habit of not eating late, as when I'd be in a show, we would be, of course, working at night. We'd be done at around ten p.m., and it was past the point where I could eat a full dinner, even after a two-hour cardio workout onstage. I'd always have trouble falling asleep and I wouldn't feel my best the next day if I ate too much. Believe me, sometimes it was hard when there would be these incredible spreads of sandwiches and burgers and pizza for us after the shows. My fellow dancers and I would avoid the food area and often have a yogurt instead, or sometimes we'd watch a movie and have some popcorn. We got so used to not eating large meals at night that we'd always eat a good, healthy breakfast, because we'd wake up hungry!

Portion Control Is Key

When I was on tour with *Burn the Floor*, one of my favorite locations was Monte Carlo. It wasn't just being on the Riviera and watching the super-rich locals with awe. No, it was waking up every morning to the delicious aroma of the wonderfully hot and crusty French baguettes and the even more delectable array of French cheeses that tempted me out of the hotel. It was impossible not to indulge in my all-consuming love for cheese, and I soon found that I was putting on a bit of weight, even though we were working so hard on the show. Worse, what I was eating was sometimes making me feel sluggish during our performances. Not that the audience knew it—but I knew it.

The simple solution was portion control. That way, I could eat my favorite cheeses—but only in small quantities. Fortunately, the local bistros served food in European-size portions, which are way smaller than American ones. My eye quickly adjusted to the portions, and I found myself full. I know that if I'd gone to the *fromageries* on my own, it would have been much more difficult not to succumb!

It is quite hard to realize the actual volume of food you're eating when it's automatically supersized for you. If you thumb through a cookbook from

Cheryl Burke Talks About How She Eats

I don't believe in diets. I've been on every single diet you can think of, and I don't think a diet is going to last a lifetime. Maybe you can do it for six to eight months and then you're going to go back to the way you were eating. I try to stay as healthy as possible, but I also try to motivate myself. Honestly, most of it is what you put in your mouth!

My weight fluctuates like any other woman's. I have more of a curvy body than the other professional dancers I was with on *Dancing with the Stars*. I went through "fat shaming" in the press about five years ago, and Kym would help me get motivated to work out and eat healthy, but I also feel like the pressure in Los Angeles and living in this kind of lifestyle is ridiculous. I've always said that being a size zero is not something you should reach for; it's not real. Of course there's pressure to be at a certain weight, but honestly it really can take over your life and is extremely unhealthy. Fans who watch *Dancing with the Stars* see our bodies, but we're in extra-great shape when we're rehearsing all day long. That can be an unrealistic goal for people and what's important is that each person finds their way to "healthy."

What works for me now is that I try not to eat past a certain time, usually around seven p.m., which is five hours before I go to bed. I wake up hungry so that motivates me to eat breakfast, which for me is the most important meal of the day as it kick-starts your metabolism. Then throughout the day it's all about portion control and keeping your body fueled with the types of food it needs. I definitely need caffeine in the morning, but instead of coffee I choose to drink caffeinated green tea, which also has detox properties.

As for weaknesses, I'm not a sugar addict—I'm a carbs addict! I like chips and salt and pizza and French fries. I say if you're going to do it then have a cheat meal once a week and eat it in the morning, or at least before two p.m. That way you can burn off a lot of it as the day goes by.

Carson Kressley on Diet and Portion Size

Before the show, my typical diet was lots of protein, tons of good-quality fresh fruits and vegetables, and even pasta for lunch—never for dinner. (Although my weakness was always French fries and champagne!) I also started each day with a glass of warm water with a tablespoon of honey and white vinegar. I really think it cleanses your system each morning, making it easier for your body to really utilize the foods you are giving it throughout the day. Once rehearsals started, I was burning so many calories that I could eat whatever I wanted. Wow, is that dangerous!

Now I try to keep complex carbs to breakfast only—but I live life and occasionally have them for lunch or even dinner. I do high protein/low carbs, and instead of dessert have a small piece of dark chocolate. That satisfies the urge for something sweet but doesn't have the calories or carbs of a full dessert. I never drink soda; instead, I like unsweetened tea and tons of water.

And the most important thing is to have small portions. I travel a lot and eat in hotels and restaurants all the time. The portions are usually insane. I almost always cut them in half. Take the other half home and you have another meal.

the 1960s or even the 1980s, you'll see how much smaller the quantities of food called for in recipes that fed four to six people were. Go out to eat and the plates are bigger, the glassware is bigger—even the silverware is bigger. Consumers grow used to these sizes and feel as if they aren't getting enough when served smaller sizes. It's a no-win situation for everyone.

You'll learn more in the next chapter about proper portions. My suggestion is that if you're craving a calorie-dense food like cheese—or my other weakness, French fries—go ahead and eat it. Enjoy it. Just eat much less of it. If you're eating out, ask for it to be taken off the table and wrapped up in a doggie bag. If you're at home, prepare only a small amount at a time. Serve it on a smaller plate, which will trick your eye into thinking there's more than there really is.

Another great way to exercise portion control is to try something I learned from going out with my girlfriends. Many of them are dancers, too, and as weight-conscious as I am because they have to be healthy. We always order a bunch of different things to share. Portion control allows me not to miss out. I find it's the best way to socialize without overeating—you're just having a taste and trying lots of things, and you don't have to worry about an enormous plate laden with fattening foods being set in front of you.

Recognize True Hunger and Eat When You're Truly Hungry

Sometimes when I was in rehearsals, I would be so focused on my work that I would literally forget to eat. My energy would plummet and I would get cranky. When that happened, I'd stop and eat something healthy like a banana or drink a smoothie, and I'd feel better right away.

I found out what true, absolutely visceral hunger was when I went on *Celebrity Survivor* in 2006. We were flown to the tiny island of Efate in Vanuatu, a tiny cluster of islands off the eastern coast of Australia. I was a bit nervous before the show started but I wanted to challenge myself to get out of my comfort zone (and you already know how important that is!), and I thought I could manage it. Well, was I in for a surprise!

We were given raw green bananas and yams to eat. And water to drink. But not to worry, we had a machete and a pot to cook the bananas and yams in. My team didn't exactly get off to a stellar start. When the other team won a challenge, they were given fish. We were given more raw green bananas and yams.

Now, you know by now that I eat a clean and healthy diet, and I don't eat a lot. I thought I would be okay with a minimal diet. But I wasn't. I had never been so hungry in my life. I'd push myself to get through the challenges and then collapse afterward. My energy plummeted; I was absolutely exhausted. I had terrible headaches. I was so cranky I couldn't see straight. I had the chance to bring one "luxury" item from home with me to the island. I chose one of my bedsheets, thinking it would be very adaptable to the circumstances. I could use it for shade or I could wear it as a blanket to sleep. When my team saw the sheet though, they got really excited and used it as a mat to cover the ground so we could all be more comfortable. Don't get me wrong, I'm a team player—but I was really counting on having a little taste of home with that sheet, and losing it put me over the edge. After only three days of very physical activity, with very little food and no sheet, I voted myself off the island!

And what did I eat as soon as I was back to civilization? An enormous plate of grilled fish. That's all I wanted. Lean, healthy protein. I don't think anything ever tasted so good in all my life.

This was a very powerful lesson for me. It was absolute proof of how harmful calorie-restrictive diets are for you. They make you feel so awful that you can't possibly continue on them. No wonder they don't work. You need to eat a balanced diet of real food, every day!

Sometimes You Think You're Hungry but You're Really Just Thirsty

I have to confess that over the years I've been very bad about drinking water, and I don't know why! Your body is about 60 percent water, and without it, you won't survive longer than two or three days. It keeps all

Florence Henderson on Her Typical Diet

I try to eat clean and healthy. I do enjoy a cocktail or wine with dinner, but I eat a lot of salads. In the morning I'll have fruits like blueberries and banana with almonds. Sometimes I'll make a smoothie using kale and blueberries or other fruit. Lunch is usually a salad, with avocado, cheese, zucchini, and tomato. I'll use fresh lemon juice as a dressing. I love greens so much my husband used to say I eat weeds! Typically, I don't eat red meat, so for dinner I'll have chicken, turkey, or fish. I really focus on having small portions. My weakness is Italian food—pasta with chopped clams and margherita pizza are my favorites—but it's all about moderation.

One of my favorite tips is that I take two teaspoons of apple cider vinegar every day, as well as a probiotic and vitamins E and D. It's good for my digestion and helps to balance my body.

your organs functioning and it makes your skin look fresh. Even when I was working up a sweat all day, I really had to push myself to get enough.

According to the Mayo Clinic, we should be drinking at least eight glasses of fluids a day. Water, of course, costs almost nothing (and no, you do not need those overpriced bottled waters!) and has zero calories. Everything you drink (milk, juice, soda, smoothies, alcohol, coffee, and tea, etc.) can be counted as part of your fluid intake, but water is best. You need to drink more when you exercise a lot, when you sweat in hot and humid weather, when you're ill, and when you're pregnant or breast-feeding.

I am much more conscious of my water intake now, and one of the ways for me to stay properly hydrated is to always start my day with a cup of hot water with lemon. I got into this great habit when I was touring with *Dancing with the Stars*, because it was easy to make in my hotel room. And then I drink it all day. I find it much more satisfying than cold water, and lemon is a wonderful food for purifying your blood and helping your liver do its detox work.

So next time you think you're hungry, have a glass of water or a cup of hot tea instead. Or make one of the amazing antioxidant tonics in chapter 5. I love making delicious anti-inflammatory concoctions of water with different ingredients like cucumber, lemon, and pomegranate. They're so yummy and have almost no calories or added sugar. Sip it slowly. If you're still hungry, then eat! If you're not, enjoy your drink . . . and then have another one.

But Be Sure Not to Drink Your Calories!

It is very easy to underestimate how calorie-dense some drinks are. An extra-large latte with whipped cream on top can contain enough calories for an entire meal, but the only nutrition comes from the milk (along with a ridiculous amount of fat and sugar from the whipped cream!). Smoothies and fresh juices are extremely high in calories, too. They may contain healthy ingredients, but watch next time you order one at a juice bar. See how many pieces of fruit get pulverized—it's far more than you could possibly eat in one sitting.

I loved making green juices that were primarily veggies when I was on *Dancing with the Stars*, but I still had to watch what I was putting in them.

Do Cleanses Work?

I must confess that sometimes, when I know I have a shoot and I want to look extra lean, I do a very short juice cleanse. I might stay on it for a day or two—never more than three—and then go right back to eating my normal diet. Cleanses are only good for a very short fix for a very specific situation, like a shoot or a special event. They don't work for normal weight loss, and they certainly don't work when you're trying to establish good eating habits, because any weight you can lose so quickly is water weight, and you'll go right back to where you were before you started the cleanse. Do calorie-restrictive cleanses for longer periods, and your metabolism actually slows down in response (to conserve energy), which means you may gain more weight if you go back to your regular diet and don't keep up your workout routine.

A lot of performers I know secretly drink 3 Ballerina Tea. It's marketed as a weight-loss tea, but its primary ingredient is senna. Senna is FDA-approved as a laxative for temporary constipation. I tried this tea, and let me tell you, you need to be near a bathroom after you drink it! It does flush you out, but, like a cleanse, it's a quick fix that has nothing to do with real weight loss. Furthermore, laxatives can be very dangerous, as the more you use them, the more you need them. And here's the catch—laxatives only work on the waste that's in your large intestine. Your food has already been digested and metabolized in your stomach and small intestine—which means the calories have already been processed before they get to the area where the tea is going to do its explosive job! You aren't actually losing real weight. You're just losing waste. And as soon as you eat again, your body will process it and get rid of it!

The moral of this story is these short-term fixes won't reward you. While you may see results immediately, in the long run a diet philosophy focused on clean eating along with a variety of exercises is a much wiser approach.

They were a treat—not a meal replacement. So I would recommend that you cut way down on sugary drinks. It's especially important to avoid all sodas, because even diet drinks trick your body into thinking you've just had something sugary, with dire results. Your body releases insulin anyway in response to this misperceived intake of something sweet; you get a blood sugar spike, which then quickly crashes down; and you're suddenly starving. This is why people who drink a lot of diet sodas often can't seem to lose any weight. (I'll discuss blood sugar more in chapter 3.) Stick to water, tea, tonics, and coffee with just a little nonfat or low-fat milk in it. Once you cut back on sugary drinks, you'll lose your taste for them. And you'll be able to eat so much more nutritious and hunger-satiating food instead.

My friend Cheryl Burke always reminds me to eat my calories. She had a trainer that recommended she eliminate sugar if she was going to have a cocktail. Instead of the fruity margarita drinks, stick to red wine, or club soda with lime and lime juice. Can you believe a margarita could have 475–500 calories? Definitely not worth it in the long run.

Watching What You Eat When You Travel Is Hard!

When I first came to the States I was so excited about diners. Yes, diners—what you Yanks call greasy spoons! We don't have them in Australia, and I'd seen them so often in movies or on TV shows and was longing to eat in one. When I finally sat down in Denny's and discovered grilled cheese sandwiches, proper French fries, tuna melts, hash browns with breakfast, and good old cheeseburgers, I was in heaven. (Jerry Springer and I often had long discussions about his favorite topic—cheeseburgers! I would use them as a bribe to get him to practice more. Once in a while, they'd smell so good that I'd join him for a burger break, and I deeply regretted it when back rehearsing on the dance floor!) And don't get me started on my favorite breakfast: a peanut butter and jelly sandwich on white bread. I thought it was the best thing in the world!

Another partner of mine, business mogul and *Shark Tank* star Mark Cuban, introduced me to my first American hot dog at a baseball game in Chicago and I surprised myself by loving it. I drank my first beer there, too. I know, it was so un-Australian of me—I'm more of a champagne kind of girl—but I don't think they served Moët at the game!

I also remember when I was about thirteen, and my dance school went for a performance in Japan. My parents came with and we stayed with a host family for a week. My mum impressed on me how important it was to be polite—which meant at least trying to eat the food our hosts were providing for us. She said this even while knowing that there are certain textures I really can't tolerate, like runny eggs (or, years later, as I discovered, escargots). So, I did my best. I ate things that I'd never eaten before and I even liked them. I was so proud of myself . . . until the host mother put down a plate of eel. I looked at it. I just couldn't. My mother gave me the eye. I tried. I just couldn't do it! And our host mother was so kind and thoughtful at the obvious distress on my face that she went out later that day and bought cereal and bread and orange juice to make me a Western breakfast the next morning. I knew it cost her a fortune and I was so touched. Every time I eat sushi now, I think of her and what my face must have looked like when I saw that eel!

I knew I had to be very careful about what I ate on the road, or I would pay for it with sluggish performances and weight gain. It can be very difficult, because you're not in your home and you're not able to cook your own food, so you can't possibly know if there are hidden calories in whatever you're eating (chicken cooked in lots of butter or oil, for example, or a rich salad dressing touted as low calorie). Sometimes, it would be extra hard, because they had great catering for us on the road. They would do their best to be considerate and bring us local specialties wherever we went, which meant a lot of fried chicken in the South that always smelled incredible. Or there would be trays of cakes—I don't know why they'd do that to dancers! Maybe I would have a bite, but I was very diligent about sticking to my usual meals of grilled chicken or salmon and lots of grilled or steamed veggies, with any sauces on the side. I'd just try to eat whatever were the healthiest-looking foods, and they always had lovely arrangements of sliced veggies and cut fruit, so that helped a lot. I never opened the minibars and I rarely ordered from room service. If I could, I'd go to the local grocery store and get some Greek yogurt and fresh fruit.

I also had to be careful about my trigger foods. That can be some-thing you particularly love—something that might even be good for you—but you know it is going to trigger a negative reaction, like bloat-ing or gas or a crummy feeling. For me, it's dairy. As you know already, cheese is my weakness. Milk always made me feel funny, even as a child, so I usually didn't drink it; cheese never bothered me in that way. But I forgot all about that funny feeling because the lattes in America are so delicious. I got into the unwise habit of drinking vanilla lattes all day, and finally, when I was complaining about how heavy and sluggish I was feeling to some of my dancer friends, someone said, "I think it's the milk." Of course it was! Out went the lattes. I lost five pounds very quickly and regained my energy. Still, staying away from them isn't easy!

As long as you know what your triggers are, you can avoid them or try to replace them with something you react better to.

Sometimes We All Need a Bit of Comfort Eating . . . and Sometimes We Need to Say No

Everyone has those nothing-has-gone-right days where all you want to do is curl up into a ball, veg out on a comfy sofa, watch some silly show or tear-jerking movie on TV, and nibble on some comfort food. I've had plenty of those days when I've been on the road, in a strange city, and I get back to my hotel room and am exhausted and missing my family, friends, and home. That's when I could easily ring up room service and eat every morsel of a cheeseburger or French fries on the plate, or call a local fast-food place to deliver some junk food and scarf it down to make myself feel better.

I know, of course, that comfort eating is just a temporary fix for whatever is ailing me. There are three things you can do when the urge hits. The first is to get up and get moving—which might be the last thing you want to do at that moment, but it can end up being the best for you. Go for a walk. Call up a trustworthy friend and talk it out while you're walking. Or do some other form of exercise. You'll be concentrating on your movement and it will make you feel better.

The second is to find a stress buster that you know will make you

Tips for Eating on the Road from Jessica Raffa,

Dancer on *Burn the Floor* and the Australian Version of *Dancing with the Stars*

Wow, eating on the road! Where can I start? Where didn't we eat!

Being a young seventeen-year-old away from home for the first time in America, I wanted to try everything. From the Cheesecake Factory to Denny's, we ate wherever we could find a decent meal. I think I went a little overboard on my first tour, as when I arrived home at the airport my family didn't recognize me. Ha!

In addition, I've always had issues finding the right foods to eat as I suffer from fructose and lactose malabsorption. I was only recently diagnosed, so while I toured with *Burn the Floor*, I couldn't understand why my tummy would bloat so much after eating just a few bites of an apple or drinking a few sips of milk. Now I know, so I avoid certain types of foods; it's difficult as many foods contain both.

Fortunately, I soon learned how to eat healthily on the road and actually became very body-conscious. It is probably a lot more difficult to do when you're touring around the world, but avoiding bad carbs and eating protein keeps you full and gives you the energy you need to perform.

feel better. Do something active or engaging that will take your mind off your troubles and your cravings. Run a hot aromatherapy bath that smells divine and have a long, soothing soak. Read that book everyone's been talking about. Play a game with your kids. Finish a task you've been putting off as you'll be so happy with yourself when it's done. Do anything at all that makes you feel good.

The third is, go ahead and have that comfort food. Occasionally. Sometimes I really need it. I will eat some French fries or a chocolate bar. Sometimes I will eat it all and go for more. Sometimes I will eat just a few bites and then push it away so I won't be tempted to eat more later!

But then, instead of beating myself up about what I just ate, I realize I ate it because I needed it and I enjoyed it. No big deal. It's done; time

Some of My Favorite Things to Eat

- For protein, I like grilled chicken; quinoa patties, which are very low in fat; and turkey burgers. I love cheese on top but instead of a bun, I'll use lettuce.

- For veggies, I love to make sweet potato fries by slicing them up and roasting them in a hot oven. I also like spaghetti squash and beets.

- For fruits, I love watermelon, all kinds of berries, kiwi, papaya, and passion fruit.

- For snacks, I go for plain Greek yogurt with manuka honey, which is local to New Zealand and full of nutrients and flavor. For crunchy things I eat almonds, although you can quickly eat a lot and they're calorie dense, so I stick to a handful. Watermelon and feta cheese is one of my favorite combinations of sweet and savory for a snack; proper feta is made from sheep's milk, so it doesn't affect me like dairy cheeses, and for some reason it pairs really well with the melon. Go figure! But it's very filling and satisfying.

to move on. And—here's the kicker—I know that I will work extra-hard tomorrow to burn it off.

I know how hard it can be to say no to tempting foods, or to friends or relatives or colleagues who are pushing you to try something when you're summoning all your willpower to refuse it. You need to stick up for yourself and have the courage to say no. It's really hard. I am a people-pleasing kind of person, and I never want to let anyone down or unwittingly hurt their feelings. But I know what is best for me and my body, and I've realized that saying no and sticking to it is extremely empowering.

Don't let yourself get stuck in the moment when you're eating something you know you shouldn't be eating. Don't call yourself names and don't punish yourself. Accept the fact that you're human and you have needs, and move on. Tomorrow will be a better-choices and a better-eating day!

Now that you know why I eat the way I do, let's take a look at the essentials of the 5-6-7-8 Diet Plan, and see how well it will work for you.

With my dog, Lola.

(3)

The 5-6-7-8 Diet Plan

As my career has shifted away from dancing 24/7, I am very aware that I can't eat what I used to eat. When I was performing nonstop, my weight remained stable even when I was on the road and being faced with tempting treats after every show. Now I have to remain vigilant and smart about what I eat. This allows me to stay healthy and not put on weight. I've adapted the best of what I've learned as a dancer into a realistic diet plan that is simple and easy to follow—and it works for me. This is what forms the basis of the unique 5-6-7-8 Diet Plans in this book. And it will work for you, too.

Why This Plan Is Different—and Why It's So Simple and Successful

Dancers hear the 5-6-7-8 cue and they're ready to go. Let me transform this for you into the right way to eat every day:

5 Servings of protein

6 Colors of the rainbow

7 Anti-inflammatory foods

8 Glasses of water

Why will the 5-6-7-8 plan work so well? It's due to its ideal balance of lean proteins and colorful fruits/vegetables, supported by proper hydration and the promotion of anti-inflammatory properties to reduce swelling and bloating. It has been designed to balance your blood sugar and insulin levels, fueling your body with protein and other nutritious whole (not processed!) foods five times throughout the day—all while ensuring you're managing your portion control, which we already know is key.

Let's take a look at this program in much more detail.

5 Servings of Protein

Protein is an essential nutrient found in food. You can't live without it. It's needed for the minute-by-minute regulation and maintenance of your body, to help keep your immune system functioning, to build and maintain muscles and bones, to help rebuild muscle after the wear and tear that occurs during workouts, and to minimize fatigue.

Every protein contains components called amino acids, and there are twenty-two different ones. Depending on which amino acids a protein contains, it is either complete, with all nine of the essential amino acids your body is unable to produce on its own, or incomplete, which means it needs supplementation from other proteins found in food. This explains why different diets are known to feature food combinations, such as rice and beans, that together supply all the essential amino acids you need.

Protein is found in animal as well as plant-based sources, as you can see in the chart below. The most common animal sources are meat, fish, poultry (including eggs), and dairy. The most common plant sources are soy, nuts, legumes, beans, grains, and some vegetables, some fruits, and seaweed (yes, even veggies and fruit can contain protein, which is something those following a vegan diet soon learn!).

This information is based on the USDA National Nutrient Database. Numbers have been rounded to make them easier to follow.

1 ounce almonds	6g
2 tablespoons peanut butter	8g
1 cup peas	8g
1 cup lentils	18g
1 cup chickpeas	15g
1 cup edamáme	17g
1 cup quinoa (cooked)	8g
1 slice sprouted-grain bread	4g
1 whole egg	6g
1 cup Greek yogurt	15g
1 ounce hard cheese	7g
4 ounces salmon	23g
4 ounces chicken breast (skinless)	26g
4 ounces beef (lean cut)	26g

Many people have no idea how much protein they actually need, and they tend to vastly underestimate it (which can lead to muscle loss and severe fatigue) or overestimate it (which can lead to weight gain, as many protein sources are calorie dense). The average adult should eat between forty-one and sixty-one grams of protein every day. Look at the chart and you can see how easy this is to do. If you have a cup of yogurt for breakfast, a serving of chicken for lunch, and a serving of fish or meat for dinner, you are well within the normal range. And this doesn't include snacks!

There is an extremely important reason why you should eat five servings of protein every day, and be sure to include some protein-rich food at every meal and snack, and it has to do with the release of insulin. This is what regulates your blood sugar and your appetite. I'll discuss this in detail in the section on carbohydrates on page 62, but for now, realize that eating protein on its own does not trigger an insulin release. Pairing protein with carbohydrate-rich foods slows down the absorption of sugar from your stomach into your bloodstream, which helps keep your blood sugar from skyrocketing and tends to ward off future cravings. Also, whenever you eat protein during your meal, it helps satiate you faster than carbohydrates. It slows down the digestion process, making you feel fuller longer. You've probably never seen anyone binge on turkey like you would see someone binge on crackers or cookies!

Digesting protein actually helps burn more calories, too. The "thermic effect of food" (TEF) is the energy we use to digest food into the small components that can be processed and absorbed into the bloodstream and then shunted to the cells where they're needed. Protein has a higher TEF compared to carbs and fat, meaning you're actually burning more calories to process protein than to process the other two.

That's why eating protein throughout the day is a good thing. You don't want surges of insulin and out-of-control blood sugar, because this is what creates a compulsive need for junk food—and the kind of weight gain that often leads to obesity and type 2 diabetes. It's why eating a typical sugary breakfast without much protein can leave you starving a mere hour or two later.

In addition, the kind of protein you want to eat is lean and clean. This means low in fat, from sources like skinless chicken breasts, all fish, Greek yogurt, and certain cuts of meat. Whenever possible, you should also try to eat meat or poultry that is grass-fed and organic, because this means it hasn't been tainted with pesticides and hormones that can, over time, have a negative effect on your health.

6 Colors of the Rainbow

Who wants a bland and boring diet with plates full of bland and boring beige, white, and brown foods? Not me! And not you, I'm sure. The more colorful your food, especially green leafy vegetables, the more nutrient-dense it is. Once you start eating foods from all colors of the rainbow, you'll wonder how you ever lived without them!

Look at the average American meals. For breakfast, many people eat a bowl of cereal or a bagel or roll or pastry. Or they eat a plate of fried eggs with home fries and toast. What color are they? For lunch, most people eat a sandwich or pasta. What color are they? For dinner, most people eat a sandwich or pasta or potatoes or rice, along with some meat or other protein. What color are they?

That's right: they're beige, white, and brown—and this means they're lacking in many nutrients, vitamins, minerals, and fiber. (There are a few exceptions, of course, and I'll discuss them on page 63.) These foods are simple carbohydrates. They are often processed foods made from white wheat flour and white sugar, or they are white rice and white potatoes. They are the basic components of fast food, junk food, and fattening, unhealthy food.

One point you need to know, however, is that your body needs carbohydrates just as it needs protein and fat. That's because your brain needs them as fuel so it can function. Once carbohydrates are processed, the fuel they provide is shuttled to your muscles in the form of glycogen.

Vegetables and fruits are carbohydrates—the good kind! An apple or squash is a simple carbohydrate, but it's a natural, unprocessed one that is consumed by your body in a much different way than processed simple carbohydrates like white flour and white sugar. So when people say they don't want to eat carbs, what they actually mean is they don't want to eat junk carbs that trigger weight gain.

UNDERSTANDING BLOOD SUGAR

Whenever you eat carbohydrates your body immediately starts to break them down, starting in your mouth as your saliva gets to work. By the time they get to your stomach, your pancreas—the organ in your body responsible for the production and release of insulin (the hormone that regulates the amount of sugar in your blood)—is already at work. Any sugar you eat, in whatever form, is broken down in your digestive tract until it is converted into glucose. It is then shuttled out of your digestive tract to your blood—this your blood sugar.

If you have a blood test measuring your blood sugar levels, it will be assessing the amount of glucose circulating in your bloodstream to provide immediate energy to cells to keep your body functioning. Glucose is converted to glycogen so it can be used by your muscles. The remaining glucose is used by other cells. If there is an excess of glucose, it can't be removed. It has to be stored in your cells for future use, where it will be leveraged for fuel. But it's not stored as glucose—it's stored as fat.

Bear in mind that a well-balanced blood sugar level is crucial to your overall fitness and well-being. It balances your hormones, triggers your body to burn stored fat, and regulates your metabolism to help you lose weight. So, yes, you need insulin to be released because without it, your body doesn't know to shuttle the glucose to your muscles and cells. (Type 1 diabetics, whose bodies don't naturally produce insulin, must inject it whenever they eat, or they will suffer serious health consequences and may be at risk for death.) But too much insulin is bad and causes weight gain.

When you eat a meal or snack that contains a mixture of good carbohydrates, good fats, and protein, it is easier for your blood sugar to remain balanced. Protein-rich foods are low on the glycemic index, which is what measures the fluctuations in a healthy person's blood sugar after eating a food containing carbohydrates. Foods that raise blood sugar quickly have a higher ranking on the glycemic index scale of 1 to 100 than foods that raise blood sugar slowly. As you learned in the section above on protein, foods that contain only protein, or protein and fat, have little or no immediate impact on blood glucose levels. This is why eating protein at every mealtime will lower the glycemic load of whatever you've ingested.

If, on the other hand, you eat a meal high in junk or processed carbohydrates, your insulin release is high. Your body goes into alert mode trying to manage the blood sugar spikes, because it can't break down all that glucose at once. It needs to get the blood sugar levels back down to normal. So what happens? Even more insulin gets released. This tells your brain that it needs nutrients. This tells your stomach to start growling. This makes you insatiably hungry.

If, in response to these cravings, you eat high-carb foods that are at the top of the glycemic index, you'll just get another insulin release, and the vicious cycle will start all over again. You are setting yourself up for endless blood sugar spikes and crashes. The excess glucose gets stored as fat. You get even hungrier. You start gaining weight and you can't understand why—how could having just a whole-grain bagel with a smear of low-fat cream cheese and a latte for breakfast make you crave another one? Because it's a sugar overload.

Typically, this happens around eleven a.m. and around three p.m., when your body has finished its initial processing of what you ate for breakfast and lunch. If you eat simple carbs made with white flour and sugar, they are digested quickly, far more so than if you eat whole grains such as steel-cut oats, or brown rice, or a pseudo-grain such as quinoa, which need a lot of chewing and contain a lot of fiber.

When you start following the 5-6-7-8 Diet Plans, you will no longer have such drastic blood sugar spikes and crashes, and the cravings for carbs will, literally, disappear. The combination of protein and complex carbs causes a slower release of blood sugar within your system. You won't need as much insulin. Your digestive system will be functioning properly. Your brain and muscles won't be screaming for fuel. And this is when you'll really see the pounds come off!

Ironically, if you eat foods that don't contain enough sugars for your body's optimal functioning, you can also start gaining weight in a hurry. That's because low blood sugar levels cause your body to go into what's called "starvation mode." This is where it starts to burn your lean muscle instead of your stored fat—because you don't have enough stored fat!—and it makes you need fewer calories to keep yourself alive. As soon as you go back to normal eating, your body doesn't recognize that, and your metabolism stays low, meaning that if you eat the same amount of calories as before the starvation mode, you will put on the pounds! It's a double whammy to your system and your diet.

Beware High-Fructose Corn Syrup!

Fructose is the sugar that naturally occurs in fruit—what makes it so sweet and delicious. Naturally occurring fructose is not bad for you; on the contrary, when you eat an entire piece of fruit, you're not only getting the natural fruit sugar but all the micronutrients and fiber your body needs. (This is why it's so much better to eat whole fruit and not guzzle a lot of fruit juice!)

High-fructose corn syrup, on the other hand, is one of the worst things in the world to eat or drink. It is derived from the sugars in corn, and it is highly processed and concentrated. Food manufacturers use it in countless products as a sweetener because it is extremely inexpensive. It is no coincidence that the obesity problem in America started to get out of control when high-fructose corn syrup—which contains anywhere from 50 to 90 percent fructose, a concentration far higher than what would ever be found in an apple or ear of corn!—became so prevalent in packaged foods. Not only is it junk sugar, but it causes high blood pressure, and the more it builds up in your liver, the more it can increase the production of blood lipids (or blood fats) and increase your risk of fatty liver disease, insulin resistance and metabolic syndrome, and type 2 diabetes.

So you should always avoid any item that includes this in its ingredient list. It is the primary sweetener of fruit drinks, non-diet sodas, sweetened yogurt, and baked goods. It is also often added to products that don't really need it, like peanut butter, sauces, and salad dressings. Always read the label!

THE IMPORTANCE OF ANTIOXIDANTS AND MICRONUTRIENTS

Rainbow-colored fruits and veggies are not only low in calories—that's because their water content is high—but they contain vital compounds called antioxidants, as well as micronutrients, which are essential vitamins and minerals and other compounds. This is what makes them effective fighters against cancer, cell damage, heart disease, and type 2 diabetes.

Antioxidants are compounds that help fight against free radicals. Whenever your body produces the energy it needs to stay alive, free radicals are the by-product. How so? Because during the energy-making process, molecules are released that are missing an electron. This is called oxidation. The molecule basically goes berserk in search of an electron to replace the missing one, and it does this by poaching an electron of another molecule in a self-perpetuating cycle. Left unchecked, free radicals can damage, prematurely age, or even kill your cells. Enter the antioxidants to put this cycle to a halt.

Free radicals are not only created internally. They're dumped on all of us every day through any toxic substances, such as air pollution, cigarette smoke, and petrochemicals. If you eat a lot of junk food, that will exacerbate your body's stress in fighting them off. A diet rich in vibrantly colored foods loaded with antioxidants will always be your best and more effective defense.

THE VITAL IMPORTANCE OF FIBER

One of the reasons for the obesity epidemic is because people often don't eat enough fiber-rich foods. Foods that are colorful all contain fiber; many foods that are white and beige are either devoid of fiber or contain very little.

Fiber is what helps you feel full. It's what you need to keep your digestive system functioning normally. Nonsoluble fiber can't be digested and so it passes in bulk through your intestines and you quickly get rid of it! (That's why fiber is so low calorie.) Without it, you will become constipated and put yourself at risk for intestinal problems if your waste is not excreted regularly. A diet lacking in fiber also puts you at a greater risk for colon cancer.

So it's as important to eat fiber-rich foods throughout the day as it is to eat protein. When your body is adjusting to the 5-6-7-8 Diet Plan, you might find yourself in the bathroom more often—and that's great! It means your digestive system is hard at work and you are absorbing the calories you need and excreting what you don't rather than storing them as fat.

THE BEST RAINBOW-COLORED CARBS TO EAT

Purple/Blue
Key Nutrients
Anthocyanins and proanthocyanins, antioxidants associated with keeping the heart healthy and the brain functioning optimally.

Go For
Blueberries, blackberries, Concord grapes, currants, figs, plums, purple grapes
Eggplant, purple cabbage, purple carrots, purple potatoes, radicchio

Green
Key Nutrients
The cruciferous vegetables, like broccoli, Brussels sprouts, cauliflower, green cabbage, and kale, contain compounds called indoles and isothiocyanates, which may help prevent cancer by amping up the production of enzymes that clear toxins from the body.

Noncruciferous vegetables and fruit are sources of the carotenoids lutein and zeaxanthin. These are strongly linked to a reduced risk of cataracts and age-related macular degeneration, the leading cause of preventable blindness in developed countries.

Go For
Avocados, green grapes, kiwis, green apples, honeydews, limes
Arugula, asparagus, broccoli, broccoli rabe, Brussels sprouts, green beans, green cabbage, celery, cucumbers, endive, leafy greens, leeks, lettuce, kale, okra, peas, green peppers, snow peas, spinach, sugar snap peas, watercress, zucchini

Yellow

Key Nutrients

These are also good sources of the carotenoids lutein and zeaxanthin, like the green fruits and noncruciferous vegetables.

Go For

Yellow apples, lemons, pineapple
Yellow beets, corn, yellow peppers, yellow squash

Orange

Key Nutrients

Alpha and beta carotene. Your body converts these compounds into the active form of vitamin A, which helps keep your eyes, bones, and immune system healthy. They also act as antioxidants.

Go For

Cantaloupes, mangoes, oranges, papayas, persimmons
Carrots, pumpkins, sweet potatoes/yams

Red

Key Nutrient

Lycopene, a phytochemical that may help fight against breast and prostate cancer.

Go For

Red apples, blood oranges, cherries, cranberries, red grapes, raspberries, rhubarbs, strawberries, watermelons
Beets, radishes, red onions, red peppers, red potatoes, tomatoes

White/Tan/Brown

Key Nutrients

White, tan, and brown are bad when you're eating processed junk foods. But they can be great when you choose certain fruits and vegetables that contain powerful antibacterial and antifungal compounds, as well as necessary micronutrients like vitamin K. Some white foods, like garlic, onions, and the bottom part of leeks, contain allicin, a sulfur-containing compound that gives fresh garlic its burning pungency. Allicin can help protect against heart disease and can lower bad cholesterol levels, but only when eaten raw.

Go For

Bananas, Anjou pears, dates, white nectarines, white peaches
Cauliflower, white corn, garlic, ginger, Jerusalem artichokes, jicama, kohlrabi, mushrooms, onions, parsnips, white potatoes, shallots, turnips
Beans and legumes (they also contain protein)

A Few Words About Grains

You may have noticed that grains are not on the list—yet!

The best grains to eat are whole and have been minimally processed. That includes grains like quinoa, steel-cut oats, spelt, barley, and buckwheat; to a lesser extent, whole wheat and other whole-grain flours like rye; and brown rice. Processed or refined grains are milled to remove the bran and germ from the kernels—which removes much of the fiber and needed micronutrients. Sometimes, the micronutrients—such as magnesium, potassium, selenium, and B vitamins—that are removed during the refining process are replaced; these products are then called enriched. It is impossible, however, to replace any lost fiber.

The reason you want to cut back on non–whole grains is that when these carbohydrates are eaten, your body very quickly breaks them down into glucose, and they trigger excessive levels of insulin. All processed grains are high on the glycemic index, which is never a good thing. So if you like to eat instant oatmeal in the morning because you believe it's healthy, the fact is that the processing of the oats to allow them to cook quickly turns them from a whole grain into a simple carbohydrate that is rapidly converted to glucose. Steel-cut oats, as you will soon discover once you start to eat them, take much longer to cook and are extremely filling. That's because they need little processing before being sold to you and are filled with fiber. Plus they're delicious! (I never eat regular oatmeal anymore because steel-cut oats are so much tastier.)

Whole-grain carbohydrates, on the other hand, are broken down more slowly due to their higher fiber content. This not only allows your body to process them more efficiently but makes you feel full faster. That's why you may not be able to finish a whole sweet potato, which is loaded with fiber, and still be full, but a whole bag of highly processed sweet potato chips, which contain much less fiber, can disappear in a

Do You Really Need Vitamin and Mineral Supplements?

After getting the go-ahead from my doctor, I started taking a good multivitamin and mineral supplement every day. Depending on your diet, your doctor may also recommend that you take certain vitamins or minerals. I think taking a multivitamin is a great way to ensure that you're not missing out on any of the key vitamins, minerals, and micronutrients that you need to function optimally. This is especially important for women who might have low levels of iron or vitamin D, especially if they are super active, pregnant, or breast-feeding.

That said, this brings me to a very important point. You should never, ever self-diagnose your health. Even if you're in great shape and brimming with energy, you should have an annual checkup with your physician, who can test your vitamin, mineral, and cholesterol levels, and many other health markers, with a simple blood test. (And being from Australia, where we are super sun-conscious, I know you should also have a full skin examination every year to check your moles and other skin spots!) That way, if any health issues arise, you will have a history to check against.

Dancers, who need their bodies to be in optimal condition, tend to be smart about their medical needs. Many of my friends are holistically minded and consult professional, licensed naturopaths, who give them advice about possible supplementation and which brands are the most effective. They are often told to take a probiotic supplement as well, which can help replenish the good bacteria in your intestines, which allows for proper digestion; many people are imbalanced, especially after antibiotic use, and have no idea this can make them feel crummy.

So be a smart consumer. You only have one body, and you shouldn't be feeding it anything just because you read about it online! Always consult your doctor before making any changes to your wellness practices.

flash and leave you wanting more. (White potatoes, by the way, are full of micronutrients, especially in the peel, but because they are high on the glycemic index, they aren't an ideal food.)

7 Anti-inflammatory Foods

Inflammation is a beast! And I don't mean just the kind of inflammation a dancer fears when we have swollen joints from long days in the rehearsal studio. I'm talking about chronic internal inflammation, which damages your cells. Scientists now recognize chronic inflammation as one of the primary underlying sources for many diseases, including arthritis, heart disease, cancers, autoimmune disorders, and obesity.

Inflammation is a natural occurrence in our bodies. You want it to happen when you get an injury, when your immune system's warriors, white blood cells in lymphatic fluid, swarm in to protect your body from bacteria and viruses, and allow healing to start. This is why injured areas get red and swollen. You don't want it to happen, however, when it's triggered for the wrong reasons, such as high levels of stress, environmental toxins, or a lack of exercise. It can even be triggered by exercise that's actually too intense.

Many people suffer from internal inflammation, however, due to an unhealthy diet. That's because the typical American diet is high in inflammatory foods. Over time, the excess fat and junk ingredients in these foods can damage cells enough to trigger an overly aggressive response from your body. These are the most common culprits when it comes to food-related chronic inflammation:

- Trans fats from hydrogenated oils and fried foods. They can damage blood vessels.

- Sugar, especially white sugar. This can send out molecules called cytokines, which can alter your body's immune response and wreak havoc. If you have a massive over-release of cytokines, this can actually trigger severe systemic inflammation that can in the worst cases be lethal.

- Foods made from flour: breads, cakes, cookies, crackers, etc. Processed foods containing large amounts of white flour, especially in combination with white sugar or high-fructose corn syrup, trigger excessive spikes of insulin and blood sugar—all leading to more inflammation!

- Alcohol in large quantities. Alcohol, like all substances your body perceives as toxic, is processed by your liver. Too much drinking can damage the cells in your liver, cause inflammation in that organ as well as in your pancreas, and can even cause brain damage.

- Monosodium glutamate, or MSG, is a commonly used flavor enhancer and food additive. It's become controversial, as evidence has shown that it might have inflammatory properties and cause swelling within cells or tissues. Many people report mild side effects after eating food doused with MSG, such as flushed cheeks, headaches, and sweating, although those are temporary.

- Processed vegetable oils like soybean, corn, safflower, and sunflower, especially once they are hydrogenated and turn into the worst of all fats—trans fats. Unhealthy fats can inflame arteries and lead to heart disease. They can also increase inflammation in the intestines that, over time, can cause bacteria to leak into the abdominal cavity, triggering even more local or systemic inflammation. (For more on fats, see the section on p. 71.)

- Processed meats. Scientists are studying how the saturated fat in processed meats can affect the bacteria in your gut; when this bacteria is imbalanced, inflammation can occur in the lining of your intestines, causing digestive problems.

Once you stop eating those foods regularly, your food-triggered inflammation will diminish. Adding at least seven different kinds of anti-inflammatory foods and drinks to your diet will make you feel even better. Take a look at the list below and count how many of those foods you actually eat on a regular basis. If it's below seven, it isn't enough.

The 5-6-7-8 Diet Plan includes a variety of different anti-inflammatory foods. It even includes tea recipes to drink at night to help fight cravings, too. (You will learn much more about anti-inflammatory drinks in the next chapter.) A diet with an abundance of plant-based foods and nutrients, adequate omega-3 fatty acids, and reduced saturated and trans fats is a powerful strategy to help lower inflammation. Eating these foods can help your body recover more quickly and less painfully after intense exercise as well. That's because our muscles tear during intense workouts, which increases internal swelling. Decreasing the amount of stress we put on our bodies by choosing the right foods helps us to heal as efficiently as possible.

SPICES AND HERBS

Spices and herbs are a fantastic way to fight inflammation, as they contain high doses of antioxidants and anti-inflammatory chemicals, especially the ones listed below. And they have negligible calories. Most people who eat a typical American diet don't cook with fresh spices and herbs and are missing out on taste, flavor, and powerful antioxidants. (The same goes for healthy fats and leafy greens!) Add them to your smoothies, cooking, baked goods, and even your coffee or tea.

Go For

Cayenne pepper, cinnamon, cloves, ginger, oregano, rosemary, turmeric

LEAFY GREENS

Foods like kale, collard greens, Swiss chard, and spinach all help protect against cellular damage and are therefore anti-inflammatory.

Go For

All leafy greens, particularly collard greens, kale, spinach, and Swiss chard

HEALTHY FATS

Good fats are loaded with micronutrients and are excellent at fighting inflammation.

Go For

Avocados, chia seeds, coconut, flaxseeds, hemp seeds, olives, pumpkin seeds, walnuts; eat whole or use their oils

ANIMAL SOURCES

Anything that comes from rivers or the oceans, or that feeds on grass, is a terrific source of omega-3 fatty acids.

Go For

Cod, halibut, herring, sardines, wild salmon, tuna, and grass-fed beef (this is what I eat); other good sources are anchovies, bluefish, mackerel, and trout

8 Glasses of Water

Our bodies are made up of roughly 60 percent water. We need a lot of water every day to keep ourselves functioning. Water helps regulate body temperature, allows us to excrete waste, helps reduce cravings for food, and keeps our tissues and muscles moist. And without it, your skin will look as parched as you feel!

We all know that water is good for us.

The average adult should drink about eight glasses of water every day. Part of your fluid intake will also come in the form of the coffee, tea, or other hot drinks you consume, as well as the foods you eat. Watermelon, for example, is nearly all water! Herbal teas that do not contain caffeine can also be counted toward your daily goal. (Caffeine is a diuretic, which means it makes you have to pee.) Eight eight-ounce glasses of water is sixty-four ounces of water, which is a little bit more than two liters. If you're there already, great!

Everyone's water intake needs are different, based on their weight, their muscle mass, their activity level, the outside temperature, and even the altitude. Take all of these things into consideration and listen to your thirst. Don't wait until you get too thirsty. Sip on water all throughout the day. On days where you sweat more than normal, or if you're pregnant or breastfeeding, increase your water intake.

Most people, however, are nowhere near that magic sixty-four, and they can unwittingly be suffering from chronic dehydration. Symptoms can include: bad breath, constipation, depression and mood swings, dry and flaky skin, a foggy feeling, headaches/migraines, muscle cramps, sugar cravings, and more. An easy way to see if you're dehydrated or not is to check your urine. The clearer the better. If it is atomic yellow, then you are most likely dehydrated or taking B vitamins.

Plain old tap water will help your body do the following:

- **Lose weight:** When your muscles are properly hydrated, you can walk, run, strength train, dance the tango, or do whatever form of exercise you choose longer and harder, giving you a more effective workout. In addition, water can increase your metabolic rate (the rate at which you burn calories) even while you're at rest. That's enough to make me drink more water now that I've gotten over my former bad habit of forgetting to do so!

- **Squash sugar cravings:** When our bodies are dehydrated, we tend to crave sweets even more. Whenever you feel an intense sugar craving coming on, drink a big glass of water first and wait five minutes. If it dissipates, you may have just been dehydrated!

- **Alleviate muscle cramping:** Dehydration can definitely be the root cause of some muscle cramping. You might also be deficient in electrolytes, which regulate our nerve and muscle functions. The most important electrolytes we need are sodium, potassium, calcium, and magnesium—which is why you'll see them listed on sports drinks meant to replenish them. If you suffer from muscle cramping, try upping your water intake and/or adding an electrolyte powder to your water. Another solution can be drinking natural coconut water, which is high in electrolytes as well.

- **Relieve headaches:** Headaches can be caused or exacerbated by dehydration. If you drink a lot of diuretics like coffee, soda, tea, or alcohol, your body could be excreting more water than it should, leaving you dehydrated. Drink plenty of water to prevent this from happening in the first place and cut down on your diuretics to see if dehydration is the culprit. Diet soda is one of the worst offenders, as it can trigger severe headaches and migraines. Fans of these sodas think the caffeine content might help reduce the pain, but they're actually making things worse. Switching to plain water can often diminish these headaches surprisingly quickly.

- Lighten your mood: Children who are thirsty are children who can be very, very cranky—and you know what that means! Tantrums, meltdowns, and embarrassed parents. Crankiness can also happen to adults, although it may not be so obvious. If you find yourself moody, depressed, foggy, or grouchy, experiment by drinking a lot more water than usual that day and see if your mood lightens. If so, recognize the signs of dehydration and up your regular intake.

One last note: if you are on the go and need to take your water with you, please use a BPA-free water bottle to refill throughout the day, as BPA is an industrial chemical used to make plastics, and it can leech out of the containers and into whatever you're consuming.

What About Fat?

You may have noticed by now that I haven't said much about fat! So here goes . . .

Fat is really not the enemy when you're thinking about weight loss. (If anything, that would be simple carbohydrates and sugar!) Just as you can't live without protein, you certainly can't live without fat. It's what keeps your brain functioning—and explains why those who cut fats way, way down often feel like they're in a fog or moving more slowly than usual. It's what cushions all your organs. It's what lubricates your digestive system. It's what makes your skin dewy and supple. It's what allows you to process vitamins A, D, E, and K (which are called fat-soluble vitamins for that reason!).

The healthy fat in your body is a lovely tan color. The unhealthy fat is opaque and white—it's the kind of fat you quickly want to trim off a cut of meat. Tan or brown fat is metabolically active; white fat is not. It's what gets stored in your body when you overeat. And it's what causes a whole slew of health problems, including obesity, fatty liver disease, metabolic syndrome, and type 2 diabetes.

Because fats are so important to a balanced diet, you need to be sure that you are eating the right kind, since there are good fats and bad fats.

ABOUT GOOD FATS

The good fats are unsaturated, either monounsaturated or polyunsaturated. They come from plant sources such as olive, canola, safflower, sesame, soybean, corn, and peanut oils; nuts and seeds; omega-3 eggs; and avocado. They also come from fattier kinds of fish like salmon.

Good fats help your body rebuild cells and produce needed hormones. Different oils also contain the omega-3 fatty acids EPA, DHA, and ALA. EPA and DHA are primarily found in fish, and ALA is primarily found in plants such as nuts and seeds, like flaxseed. Omega-3 fatty acids can lower your levels of blood fats and alleviate joint stiffness, and may help with depression and mood disorders.

The best good fats are: avocado, chia seeds, coconut oil, flaxseed/flax oil, hemp seeds, olive oil, pumpkin seeds/oil, and walnut oil. Although coconut oil is saturated, its fatty acid composition is unique, and it has other health benefits, so it is safer to eat than other saturated fats.

ABOUT BAD FATS

The bad fats are saturated. They are found in certain plant oils as well as animal sources. This list includes meat, including suet and lard; dairy, including butter; palm and palm kernel oil. Saturated fats are also found in any prepared or processed foods that contain trans fats, hydrogenated oils, or partially hydrogenated oils. That includes almost all fast food, junk food, baked goods, and fried foods.

The very worst of the bad fats are trans fats. They are created when hydrogen is added to a vegetable oil; food manufacturers use them because they are inexpensive, they increase shelf life, and they can improve taste—but they can also increase your levels of bad cholesterol (LDL) while decreasing your levels of good cholesterol (HDL). Just so you know, cholesterol isn't a fat. It's a sort of fatlike substance that your body must have in order to create its cells and produce some hormones. And because your body is perfectly capable of making its own cholesterol, you don't need to get it from your food, unlike certain vitamins. That's why diets high in saturated fat increase the unhealthy LDL, in turn increasing your risk for clogged arteries, heart disease, type 2 diabetes, and strokes.

You should always avoid any packaged foods that contain the words "partially hydrogenated" on the label, as that's the scientific name for trans fats. Stay away from highly processed oils (sunflower, corn, safflower, soybean, or margarine) as well.

KEEPING FAT TO A MINIMUM

This is what I like to do to manage my fat intake:

- **Avoid any solid fats.** Go for liquid vegetable oils instead. For example, sauté with olive oil instead of butter, and use canola oil when baking. The only exception for me is coconut oil. I love how it tastes (and it's also great for your skin as a moisturizer!). As you read already, although coconut oil contains saturated fat, it is one of the rare exceptions where something once thought of as unhealthy is actually good for you to use. That's because it contains no cholesterol. It also provides a quick source of energy and has been shown to help protect against infections and kill various bacteria, fungi, and viruses.

- **Use olive oil in salad dressings and marinades.** Once you start using it, you'll see that there's a tremendous variety of olive oils with distinctive colors and tastes. Making your own vinaigrette is super easy and super delicious. It makes any salad taste better! I often like to mix olive oil with lemon juice and a variety of spices to make each salad unique.

- **Select milk and dairy products that are low in fat.**

How to Clean Out Your Kitchen: What Foods Get Tossed and Why

When you start the 5-6-7-8 Diet Plan, it's important you do your homework and are prepared. This will set you up for success—and success starts at home.

So step one is to do a thorough kitchen clean-out, including your cupboards and pantry, your refrigerator, your freezers, and even your drawers. And although this isn't part of your kitchen, be sure to go through your car, as many people stash snacks and drinks there, too! You want to toss or donate any foods that will distract you from your goals.

Instead, what you should aim to do is line your shelves with whole foods. This means they are minimally processed and contain only one primary ingredient, like fresh, frozen, or canned (no sugar added) fruit and vegetables; nuts; protein sources like chicken breasts or canned salmon; and my favorite, Greek yogurt. It's higher in protein than regular yogurt, and it's very filling.

SUGAR IS EVERYWHERE—AND HERE'S HOW TO FIND IT

As you know, any excess sugar in our diet that is not metabolized or burned off will be stored in your cells as fat. Of course, we also all know how important it is to limit the amount of sugar we eat—but it's not realistic to try to avoid it altogether. Sometimes I just need a piece of chocolate! So here are the best tips for helping you spot and get rid of sugars, either hiding or in plain sight:

- When reading ingredients on a food label, remember that most words that end in -ose are some form of sugar. Some of the names to look for are dextrose, maltose, sucrose, fructose, glucose, galactose, lactose, and xylose. Other forms of sugar are high-fructose corn syrup, corn syrup, corn sweetener, rice syrup, dehydrated cane juice, cane sugar, fruit juice concentrate, barley malt, beet sugar, molasses, brown rice syrup, honey, maple syrup, agave nectar, coconut sugar, date sugar, evaporated cane juice, sorghum, tapioca syrup, and turbinado sugar. They're all sugar and they're all bad for you, even if they're organic.

- When reading the nutrition facts label on any food item, be sure to check how many grams of sugar per serving the food contains. First look to see how many servings the item contains; manufacturers can be sneaky, because they'll often put "two servings" on a small brownie or bottle of soda, when they know full well that you consider it to only be one serving! Anything over seven grams per serving is starting to get steep, and you may want to reconsider your choice.

- Sugar can lurk unexpected in many different foods; it's added to improve the flavor. Store-bought tomato sauces, breads, barbecue sauce, salad dressings, instant oatmeal, cereals, snack bars, protein bars, and yogurt can contain surprisingly large amounts of sugar. Some contain more sugar than a candy bar!

- When you do want to use a touch of sweetener, go with the most natural form possible, like honey or maple syrup. These contain trace minerals, and the best grades have antimicrobial properties as well.

SUGARS, REAL AND FAKE, THAT MUST GET TOSSED!

While you want to cut down on your overall sugar consumption, certain sugar-laden items can be very dangerous for your health when consumed regularly:

- **Soda:** One twelve-ounce can of cola can contain about thirty-three grams of sugar—which is the equivalent of about ten teaspoons! The dangerous amount of sugar in soda spikes blood sugar and insulin responses. Over time, this can contribute to obesity and type 2 diabetes. If that's not bad enough, most sodas contain large amounts of phosphoric acid, which not only rots teeth and gums but can accelerate aging and lead to osteoporosis by leaching calcium from your bones.

- **Foods or drinks with high-fructose corn syrup:** As you read in the sidebar on page 60, this is the sugar beloved of the food industry because it's so inexpensive. Once you start reading labels, you will likely be shocked at how many foods contain it. One of the worst culprits is juice drinks.

- **Juice:** Speaking of which, juice is nothing more than concentrated sugar, even if you squeeze it yourself. Many juice drinks are nothing more than sugar water with a tiny bit of real juice added. They're terrible for kids and terrible for you. So if you like juice, go for green juices that are primarily veggies and use only a tiny bit of fruit for sweetness and palatability. If you like bottled "healthy" juices or smoothies, be sure to read the labels. It's a consumer con when a super-expensive bottle of "green juice" has apple juice at the top of the ingredient list.

- **Candy:** Candy comes in all colors, shapes, and sizes. You know how hard it can be to just eat a little. The primary ingredient of all candy is sugar—a lot of sugar. Although a bag of sweet candies may contain less than two hundred calories, it often contains forty to fifty grams of sugar! When you want a sweet treat, have one ounce of dark chocolate instead; the darker the better. (For more about the benefits of dark chocolate, see page 85 in chapter 4.)

- **Cold cereals with either sugar or white wheat flour as the first two ingredients:** They usually contain artificial colors and preservatives, too. These highly processed pseudo-nutrients will cause an immediate insulin spike and leave you starving soon thereafter. This is no way to start your day, or to eat a snack either.

- **Packaged snack foods, like chips, pretzels, cookies, and crackers:** Again, read the labels. Sugar is usually near the top of the ingredient list, along with the trans fats and highly refined flours that can pack on the pounds. Removing these from your home will help you resist their calling. Out of sight, out of mind!

- **Artificial no-calorie sweeteners:** Your body is programmed to release insulin whenever you eat or drink something sweet. Just because these contain zero calories doesn't mean they are a healthy option. That's because these chemicals modify the way your body naturally processes sugar, making you more susceptible to overeating because you're getting the same insulin spikes even though you haven't eaten real sugar! Beware of artificial sweeteners with these names: aspartame, erythritol, isomalt, lactitol, maltitol, saccharin, sorbitol, sucralose, and xylitol.

- **Fat-free baked goods:** What is the fat replaced with? You guessed it—sugar. The calories might be slightly reduced, but don't fall for the hype. These foods are pure junk.

THE REST OF THE FOODS YOU WANT TO TOSS!

"All-Natural"

Seeing that on a package usually means one thing: you are about to get conned. All food should be all-natural, right? But poison ivy and arsenic are all-natural, too. So is snake venom. "All-natural" is often added to the front of a bag or box of junk food to make you think that what you're getting is healthy. Trust me—it isn't!

Processed Meat

Most bacon, ham, salami, sausage, and hot dogs are dangerous for your health. They are processed with a chemical called sodium nitrite, which turns the color of the meat red so it looks fresh. This chemical forms cancer-causing agents in your body—which means you're increasing your cancer risk whenever you eat them. (If you like these foods, look for meat that is nitrite-free; it will be clearly labeled on the package.)

Non-natural Peanut Butter

Nut butters are very filling and a good source of protein and healthy fats. But real peanut butter has only one or two ingredients. The first is peanuts and the second, optional, ingredient is salt. Non-natural peanut butter will include sugar and partially hydrogenated oils. These trans fats are linked to an increase in heart disease and should never be eaten, not even in moderation.

White Bagels, White Breads, and Pastries

All foods made from processed white and wheat flour should be avoided for an optimal healthy diet. Flour has a high glycemic index, meaning that it spikes your blood sugar quickly and therefore raises insulin levels. Foods made from flour have little nutritional value, and a diet high in them can lead to obesity, inflammation, and type 2 diabetes. Be sure to read labels carefully, as many foods are sold as "whole-grain" when the primary ingredient is white flour with a much smaller percentage of whole grains added. If the bread is truly whole-grain, the first ingredient will be whole-wheat flour. If other whole grains are added, such as rye, they will have "whole-grain" in front of them, too.

Deep-Fried Foods

French fries, onion rings, mozzarella sticks, and doughnuts are just some of the foods on my please-don't-eat list. Because they are fried in fat, fried foods are much higher in calories than if they were baked, steamed, or roasted. They are also dangerous, because most restaurants will use partially hydrogenated oils—the infamous trans fats—for frying and likely increase your risk of heart disease.

Your Go-To List of the Best Foods to Eat

Now that your shelves are clear, let's see what you can put on them!

PROTEIN
Chicken
Fish
Grass-fed beef
Greek yogurt
Shellfish
Tofu*

CANNED GOODS OR
TETRA PAKS
Black beans, kidney beans,
    white beans
Chickpeas
Coconut milk
Lentils
Nut milks (cashew, almond)
Stewed or whole tomatoes

PANTRY (DRIED GOODS)
Brown rice
Pasta (whole-wheat or
    gluten-free varieties)
Quinoa
Steel-cut oats

PRODUCE

Fruit
Apples
Avocados
Bananas
Berries
Lemons
Limes
Melons

Frozen produce
Beans
Berries (strawberries, blueberries,
    raspberries, blackberries)
Broccoli
Peas
Spinach

Vegetables
Lettuce
Baby carrots
Cucumbers
Celery
Baby tomatoes
Sweet potatoes/yams

*Tofu is nutritious and filling, and since it's on the bland side it works well with different sauces or in a salad with a delicious homemade vinaigrette. But because much of the tofu sold in America is made from genetically modified (GMO) soybeans that have been treated with herbicides, which I don't recommend you eat, you should only buy organic tofu that is certified and labeled non-GMO. And if you like soy milk, also look for organic brands that are non-GMO.

SNACKS

Raw almonds

Walnuts

Almond butter

Peanut butter (natural)

Pumpkin seeds

Dried fruit: cranberries, cherries,
    raisins, currants

Hummus

Dried seaweed

OILS/CONDIMENTS

Apple cider vinegar

Coconut oil

Hot sauce

Mustard

Olive oil

Tamari or soy sauce, low sodium

Walnut oil

SWEETENERS

Honey, preferably raw

Maple syrup

SPICES

Garlic (fresh and powdered)

Sea salt

Pepper

Turmeric

Fresh ginger

Cinnamon

Cayenne

DRINKS

Decaf coffee

Herbal tea

Homemade fizzy water (use a
    SodaStream machine)

Water, from the tap!

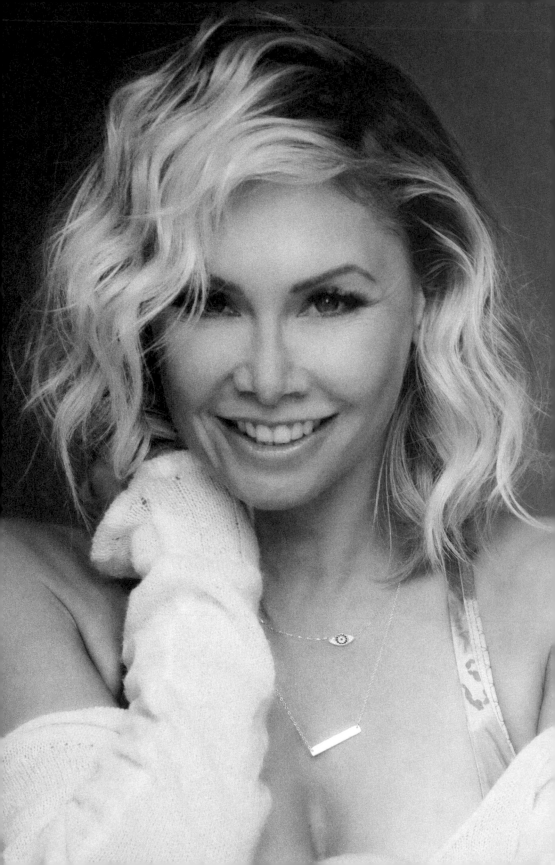

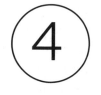

The 5-6-7-8
Fourteen-Day
Diet Plan

Are you ready to transform the way you eat? Great!

As you'll see in these diet plans, the 5-6-7-8 plan is extremely easy to follow. Just remember the basics you should include every day:

5 Servings of protein

6 Colors of the rainbow

7 Anti-inflammatory foods

8 Glasses of water

Here are more specifics:

Calorie Count

This diet plan is based on roughly fifteen hundred calories per day. But—and this is a big but!—I'd like to steer you away from worrying about calorie counting. That's because every person has a different caloric need based on their current weight, goal weight, muscle mass, and innate metabolism. If you're really amping up your workouts, you need more calories. If you're stuck on a big project at work and have less time than usual to move, eat slightly less. What's most important is to be able to gauge your true hunger and adjust accordingly. If you feel like you are eating too much, then reduce your snack portions. If you feel like you are hungry all the time, then you should increase your snack portions. Adjust slowly. Listen to your body. As you know, you have to be realistic and set attainable goals for yourself. But I can promise you that it doesn't take very much time at all to lose your taste for sugar and to adjust your portion size.

Portion Control

When I asked my former *Dancing with the Stars* partner Joey Fatone if he had any tips about portion control, this is what he said: "Wire your mouth shut!"

That made me laugh (especially because I knew he was kidding!). We all know that choosing healthy foods is key, but even the healthiest foods in excessive amounts can make us gain weight. Once you adjust your portion sizes, you will become used to eating the appropriate amount. Remember all the tricks I told you about on page 40 in chapter 2? This is the time to really take them to heart. And be sure to eat slowly! Keep these rules in mind when thinking of portion control:

- A four-ounce serving of protein is about the size of a smartphone or the palm of your hand.

- When eating grains, use the visual of a tennis ball to control your portion of these carbohydrates. This would equal about one cup. In some cases, though, you will find that your serving sizes of carbs may be slightly less than this in the meal plans.

- A serving size of food containing healthy fats, such as almond butter or avocado, can be measured by visualizing the size of a golf ball. This equals about two tablespoons.

- When eating dairy and nuts, keep in mind the size of a Tic Tac container or a shot glass. This represents a one-ounce serving.

- When making smoothies, an average serving size is no more than sixteen ounces. You already know not to drink your calories, so be careful!

- There are no limits on leafy greens and salad greens.

- There are also no limits on anti-inflammatory teas or water.

Reach for the Teakettle!

As I wrote about in the section on comfort eating (page 49) in chapter 2, nighttime is often the time when the stress of the day has gotten to you and you feel the need for comfort food. I know the feeling all too well, especially because I do have a sweet tooth, and instead of reaching for the snacks or a sweet dessert I might once have craved, I've gotten myself into the habit of drinking these delicious teas instead.

These teas are not just flavorful and satisfying. They are functional and contain potent ingredients. Not only are they anti-inflammatory, but they will aid with your digestion and fill you up with zero or few calories. As you'll see, they all have a purpose and are aptly named: Detox Tea, Anti-inflammatory Tea, Sweet Comfort Tea, and Digestion Tea.

- When you first begin the fourteen-day diet plan: Drink the Detox Tea. This will help you make the transition to a whole-foods diet, especially if you have been eating a typical American diet with a lot of processed food. I really love this tea and drink it nearly every day. Even if you aren't following my diet plan, this tea will greatly aid your digestion, especially your liver—that's the organ most responsible for your body's daily detox. It's especially helpful after a heavy or a splurge meal. The apple cider vinegar aids in digestion, green tea helps improve your metabolism, and lemon is a wonderful purifier that helps to balance out acidity in your body.

- If you are feeling sore from a workout: Drink the Anti-inflammatory Tea. The active ingredient in turmeric is called curcumin and is a well-known and powerful anti-inflammatory and antioxidant. It has been extensively studied and is often used to help those who suffer from joint and muscle pain, as it helps reduce swelling. Many dancers I know take curcumin as a supplement for just this reason.

- If you are craving sweets and/or chocolate: Drink the Sweet Comfort Tea. Cacao is high in antioxidants and magnesium, which is a mineral that is particularly good for muscle recovery. Muscle cramping can be a sign of magnesium deficiency. Also, the week before your period is a great time to have extra magnesium on hand, as your hormonal fluctuations often lead to cravings at this time—doubtless as you well know!

- If you have bloating or stomach upset: Drink the Digestion Tea. Ginger is a pungent root that is great detoxifier, an anti-inflammatory, and a stomach calmer. Many people like to take it for nausea and motion sickness as well.

The recipes for these teas can be found on pages 100 to 102 in chapter 5. Here are the ingredients you'll need to have on hand for them:

Canned light coconut milk

Cacao powder

Cinnamon

Cayenne

Green tea bags

Lemon

Honey

Apple cider vinegar

Ginger (fresh)

Ginger powder

Maple syrup

Turmeric

The Cravings Swap List

When people have cravings, they tend to fall into one of these categories: savory, crunchy, salty, or sweet. Some of those with a sweet tooth (like me!) find themselves satisfied with a piece of really good dark chocolate, which has fiber, minerals, and antioxidant properties. Eating a lot of it isn't advisable, but if you're going to indulge, go for the very best and savor it slowly.

One of the best swaps you can make—and this is in moderation only, of course—is to replace any chocolate candy bars and candy pieces with a small square of dark chocolate instead. The milk chocolate you're used to is loaded with sugar and fat, and usually not the good kind of fat, as well as other unhealthy ingredients. And we all know how hard it is to stop once you open up the packet!

Dark chocolate, especially when it has a high cacao content, has proven health benefits. That's because it contains plant nutrients called flavonoids, and these are antioxidants. They can help to lower blood pressure and help improve blood circulation. Many researchers are also investigating dark chocolate's health benefits, and some studies suggest it gives protection against heart attacks, strokes, and diabetes. Obviously, you don't want to eat a lot of it, and because dark chocolate is very dense and yet not very sweet, it's meant to be savored. But get the best-quality chocolate you can afford, as you'll be surprised at how different brands sourced from different cacao beans can taste.

And for those who love potato chips or other crunchy chips, try a pickle instead! I know it sounds a bit crazy, but when you want something salty and crunchy, a pickle (made from cucumbers steeped in brine) not only satisfies the need to bite into something but has almost no calories. Or try using a condiment like mustard on a slice of turkey, which tickles your savory taste buds and helps make the cravings disappear.

Avoid	Go For
Baked goods	Plain Greek yogurt with a swirl of honey or jam
Breakfast cereal	Steel-cut oatmeal
Candy	Cut-up dried fruit, berries, watermelon
Chocolate	Small piece top-quality dark chocolate, raw cacao nibs
Creamy desserts	Chia pudding
French fries	Baked sweet potato fries (recipe on page 119)
Mayonnaise	Plain yogurt or mashed avocado
Potato chips	Pickles
Salad dressing	Homemade vinaigrette with olive or walnut oil

The 5-6-7-8 Diet Plan: Jump-Start Your Weight Loss

We've included many delicious, nutrient-loaded, and low-calorie recipes in the next chapter, and these lists here contain many of them. It's very helpful to know what exactly to buy when you go shopping for these first two weeks, so I've also drawn up shopping lists.

You'll notice that some of the recipes repeat in the week. The reasons for that are simple: it's less time-consuming for you to double the recipes and cook up bigger batches of meals, then eat the leftovers (which is how I eat!), and this cuts way, way down on your grocery bills. Once you start cooking fresh food, I think you will be astonished at how much money you are saving. Packaged food is rarely cost-effective, and junk

Dancer Janelle Hallier's Diet Tips

Like Kym, I always remember to eat something at least every two to three hours. I never go longer than three hours without food. This is what I eat on a typical day:

For breakfast, I'll have two eggs cooked in a little bit of butter with sprouted whole-wheat toast and some sliced avocado.

For a midmorning snack I'll have a protein shake, cut-up vegetable crudités, or a green juice.

For lunch, I'll have chicken or fish with a salad. I like to keep it simple and easy and just do fresh arugula or baby spinach with tomatoes. The dressing is simple and easy, too: a splash of lemon, a splash of apple cider vinegar, a little bit of olive oil, and salt and pepper.

For a midafternoon snack, I'll choose one item from the morning snack list.

For dinner, same as lunch. Maybe I'll add different veggies to the salad.

For an evening snack, same thing—choose from the morning list.

I also have a special drink that I go for three times a day: a big glass of green tea with a squeeze of lemon and a splash of apple cider vinegar. I'll drink one first thing in the morning on an empty stomach, get ready for the day, and then eat breakfast; the next one at midday; and the last one before bed.

food always costs more than real food. If you look at a box of macaroni and cheese, for instance, the box usually weighs about six ounces—that includes the dried pasta and the fake cheese in the packet. That box usually costs at least double what a pound of dried pasta costs. You are paying a premium for the convenience of tearing open a packet of fake cheese. Then you still have to cook it and make the sauce—and if you make your own healthier version, it will not only taste so much better and be so much better for you, but it will save you a lot of money.

At the end of this section, I've included suggested meal options so you can get some ideas about how to mix and match the recipes you'll find in the next chapter.

Week 1

Monday
Breakfast: Green Smoothie
Snack 1:   Egg on a Brown Rice Cake*
Lunch: Open-faced SALT (Salmon, Avocado, Lettuce, Tomato)
                Sandwich
Snack 2:   Greek Yogurt and Berries
Dinner: Ginger Shrimp and Broccoli Stir-fry
Teatime: Your choice

Tuesday
Breakfast: Spinach Goat Cheese Scramble
Snack 1:   Apple with Almond Butter
Lunch: Arugula, Olive, and Grilled Chicken Salad
Snack 2:   Snap Peas and Hummus
Dinner: Spinach, Apple, Quinoa, and Goat Cheese Salad
Teatime: Your choice

Wednesday
Breakfast: Green Smoothie
Snack 1:   Egg on a Brown Rice Cake
Lunch: Open-faced SALT (Salmon, Avocado, Lettuce, Tomato)
                Sandwich
Snack 2:   Greek Yogurt and Berries
Dinner: Ginger Shrimp and Broccoli Stir-fry
Teatime: Your choice

---

*A rice cake made from white rice and eaten on its own is high on the glycemic index. But when paired with a healthy fat or protein, such as egg, the snack takes longer to digest and the glycemic load goes way down. I like brown rice cakes as they are made from whole grains, and are crunchy and filling. Many of the dancers I know swear by them! And if you're not crazy about eggs, then try the rice cake with a tablespoon of hummus or peanut butter, a small square of cheese like feta or tofu, or a small piece of grilled chicken or fish. What's most important is to mix the rice cake with a protein or healthy fat.

Thursday

Breakfast:	Spinach Goat Cheese Scramble
Snack 1:	Apple with Almond Butter
Lunch:	Arugula, Olive, and Grilled Chicken Salad
Snack 2:	Snap Peas and Hummus
Dinner:	Spinach, Apple, Quinoa, and Goat Cheese Salad
Teatime:	Your choice

Friday

Breakfast:	Green Smoothie
Snack 1:	Egg on a Brown Rice Cake
Lunch:	Pasta, Peas, and Pesto
Snack 2:	Greek Yogurt and Berries
Dinner:	Steak Plate with Spinach and Grilled Mushrooms
Teatime:	Your choice

Saturday

Breakfast:	Protein-Packed Pancakes
Snack 1:	Apple with Almond Butter
Lunch:	Arugula, Olive, and Grilled Chicken Salad
Snack 2:	Snap Peas and Hummus
Dinner:	Spinach, Apple, Quinoa, and Goat Cheese Salad
Teatime:	Your choice

Sunday

Breakfast:	Protein-Packed Pancakes
Snack 1:	Egg on a Brown Rice Cake
Lunch:	Pasta, Peas, and Pesto
Snack 2:	Greek Yogurt and Berries
Dinner:	Steak Plate with Spinach and Grilled Mushrooms
Teatime:	Your choice

Shopping List, Week 1

Fruits/Vegetables

Apples
Arugula
Avocados
Baby spinach
Baby tomatoes
Bananas
Berries (your choice)
Broccoli
Carrots
Cucumber
Kale
Kiwi
Lemons
Lettuce (Romaine)
Olives (Kalamata)
Onions
Portobello mushrooms
Snap peas (or sugar snap
    peas)
Tomatoes

Dairy/Eggs

Eggs
Goat cheese
Nonfat plain Greek yogurt
Parmesan cheese

Grains

Brown rice
Sprouted-grain bread
    (often called Ezekiel
    bread)
Whole-grain pasta
    (fusilli or farfalle)
Quinoa
Rice cakes (plain,
    brown rice)

Legumes

Hummus
Peas (frozen)

Meat/Fish

Chicken breast
Flank steak
Salmon
Shrimp

Nuts/Seeds

Almond butter
Pumpkin seeds (roasted)
Walnuts

Oils

Coconut oil
Olive oil

Spices/Herbs

Cinnamon
Garlic
Ginger

Miscellaneous

Apple cider vinegar
Balsamic vinegar
Baking powder
Honey (raw is best)
Maple syrup (pure)
Pesto
Stock (can be veggie,
    chicken, or beef)
Tamari (can use soy sauce
    instead)

Week 2

Monday

Breakfast:	Cinnamon Greek Yogurt Parfait
Snack 1:	DIY Trail Mix
Lunch:	Quinoa Bowl with Roasted Vegetables
Snack 2:	Edamame, Lemon, and Salt
Dinner:	Beets, Feta, and Grilled Chicken Salad
Teatime:	Your choice

Tuesday

Breakfast:	Zucchini Goat Cheese Frittata
Snack 1:	Cinnamon Chia Pudding
Lunch:	Black Bean Avocado Salad
Snack 2:	Dark Chocolate Almond Butter Balls
Dinner:	Steamed Salmon and Broccoli over Cauliflower Mash
Teatime:	Your choice

Wednesday

Breakfast:	Cinnamon Greek Yogurt Parfait
Snack 1:	DIY Trail Mix
Lunch:	Quinoa Bowl with Roasted Vegetables
Snack 2:	Edamame, Lemon, and Salt
Dinner:	Beets, Feta, and Grilled Chicken Salad
Teatime:	Your choice

Thursday

Breakfast:	Zucchini Goat Cheese Frittata
Snack 1:	Cinnamon Chia Pudding
Lunch:	Black Bean Avocado Salad
Snack 2:	Dark Chocolate Almond Butter Balls
Dinner:	Steamed Salmon and Broccoli over Cauliflower Mash
Teatime:	Your choice

Friday

Breakfast:	Cinnamon Greek Yogurt Parfait
Snack 1:	DIY Trail Mix
Lunch:	Salmon Niçoise Salad
Snack 2:	Edamame, Lemon, and Salt
Dinner:	Turkey Burger with Spicy Sweet Potato "Fries"
Teatime:	Your choice

Saturday

Breakfast:	Mocha Banana Nut Smoothie
Snack 1:	Cinnamon Chia Pudding
Lunch:	Black Bean Avocado Salad
Snack 2:	Dark Chocolate Almond Butter Balls
Dinner:	Steamed Salmon and Broccoli over Cauliflower Mash
Teatime:	Your choice

Sunday

Breakfast:	Mocha Banana Nut Smoothie
Snack 1:	DIY Trail Mix
Lunch:	Salmon Niçoise Salad
Snack 2:	Edamame, Lemon, and Salt
Dinner:	Turkey Burger with Spicy Sweet Potato "Fries"
Teatime:	Your choice

Shopping List, Week 2

NOTE: You will already have many of the staples, such as the grains, legumes, oils, and spices/herbs, on hand. It's less expensive to buy them in bulk and most of these items don't need refrigeration. Always look to buy fresh produce and meat/fish as they will taste better and contain more nutrients.

Fruits/Vegetables

Avocados

Beets

Berries (your choice)

Broccoli

Capers

Carrot

Cauliflower

Cranberries (dried)

Green beans

Lemons

Lettuce (Romaine)

Limes

Olives (Kalamata)

Pickles

Red onions

Salad greens

Sweet potatoes

Tomatoes

Yellow squash

Zucchini

Dairy/Eggs

Eggs

Feta cheese

Goat cheese

Nonfat plain Greek yogurt

Grains

Brown rice

Oats

Quinoa

Sprouted-grain bread

Legumes

Black beans (canned)

Edamame (frozen)

Meat/Fish

Chicken breast

Salmon (fresh and canned for salad)

Turkey patties

Nuts/Seeds

Almonds (raw)

Almond butter

Chia seeds

Hazelnuts

Pumpkin seeds

Oils

Coconut oil

Olive oil

Spices/Herbs

Cayenne

Chives

Cilantro

Cinnamon

Cumin

Garlic powder

Rosemary

Miscellaneous

Almond milk

Balsamic vinegar

Cacao powder

Chocolate chips (dark chocolate)

Coffee

Dijon mustard

Honey

Hot sauce

Maple syrup

The Fourteen-Day Diet Plan Options

Breakfast Options

Green Smoothie

Mocha Banana Nut Smoothie

Spinach Goat Cheese Scramble

Zucchini Goat Cheese Frittata

Cinnamon Greek Yogurt Parfait

Lunch Options

Quinoa Bowl with
    Roasted Vegetables

 Grilled Chicken Salad

Salmon Niçoise Salad

Vegetarian Salad (my favorite veggies plus
    black beans or other beans)

Pasta, Peas, and Pesto

Turkey Burger with Spicy Sweet Potato
    "Fries"

Dinner Options

Steak Plate with Spinach and Grilled
    Mushrooms

Ginger Shrimp and Broccoli Stir-fry

Beets, Feta, and Grilled
    Chicken Salad

Salmon and sweet potatoes

Energizing Snack List

Popcorn with Pumpkin Seeds
    (or pistachios)*

A Frozen Banana

Protein-Packed Pancakes

Greek Yogurt and Berries

Snap Peas and Hummus

Edamame, Lemon, and Salt

Cinnamon Chia Pudding

DIY Trail Mix

Dark Chocolate Almond Butter Balls

* You should avoid eating packaged microwave popcorn, as it is almost always loaded with trans fats, artificial colors and flavors, and a lot of chemical preservatives.

The 5-6-7-8 Maintenance Plan

Now that you've been eating so well for two weeks, how do you feel? I hope that your cravings have subsided, you're seeing some of the benefits of this life change, and you're ready to move forward.

As you transition off the weight-loss fourteen-day plan it's important you stick to the 5-6-7-8 philosophy. To get the most benefits from this program after your two-week jump-start, here's what to do:

- Remember that portion control is king. Just because your plate is full doesn't mean you need to eat it all. Cut the portions in half, share with a friend, or take the rest home for another meal.

- Depending on your lifestyle and activity level, you might want to tweak your calorie intake and add some more. The meal plans are based on your eating approximately 1,500 calories per day, which includes the two snacks. Depending on your weight loss or fitness goals, this may not be enough. To bolster that by approximately 200–300 calories per day, I recommend increasing your portion sizes only slightly. The easiest way to do that is to consume more vegetables with each meal. This will help you bolster the "colors of the rainbow" that you're eating while still increasing the healthiest types of carbohydrates. You might also want to experiment with the size of your snacks and eat a bit more protein with them.

- As you know by now, the 5-6-7-8 plan is relatively light in terms of the grains you're consuming—and I'll bet you don't miss them as much as you thought you might! That said, I know how hard it is to cut out all processed carbohydrates and grains. Just do your best to avoid them as a regular part of your diet. Don't deprive yourself of a slice of your daughter's birthday cake at her party—go ahead and enjoy it! What you've learned is to see the kind of junk carbs that make up the average diet as treats, not an integral part of your meals. So what I recommend is that as you increase your calories, you add in a few more whole grains. Have a bit more brown rice or a bigger bowl of steel-cut oatmeal. As a general rule, I almost never eat any processed carbs after lunchtime. That's because these foods cause blood sugar spikes and can make me hungry again in a short time, even after I've eaten a large meal. When that happens, I know to eat more protein for my snack as that will not trigger a release of insulin.

When I was on *Dancing with the Stars* and sharing my diet tips with my partners, and when I was devising this plan, many people asked me about what they called a cheat day, or an 80/20 diet philosophy—that's when you strive to eat as healthily as possible 80 percent of the time and eat less well for the other 20 percent. Or when you set aside a certain day of the week to eat whatever you want. I know this kind of eating works for some people. I also know that there will be times when you're going out to dinner and the bread bowl arrives, and you eat all of it. Or when you know you are going to have French fries and a bacon cheeseburger for dinner. This is a natural part of everyone's challenge with food. We're all going to have days when we just want those extra few bites. Sometimes, too, we are faced with event after event or weekends away from home—and we can't stick to our plan.

That's life!

The point of the 5-6-7-8 plan, though, is to create a sense of balance so that your cravings are limited and you get all the deeply satisfying and nutritious fuel you need. This plan will help you maintain your energy levels and keep your weight down with appropriate amounts of protein, vegetables, carbs, and healthy fats. So, sure, you may reach for the fries every once in a while—and that's okay—but you won't feel that you need them.

This is why the 80/20 philosophy doesn't work for me, because you don't want to give yourself a day off—or a cheat day. That implies that it's okay to waver in your philosophy. And how I have taught you to eat in this book is how you'll want to eat—for life!

If you're working to make a change in your life and in your overall health and fitness, then it's important you stay motivated and committed to the plan. Once you've achieved your goal and you're looking to maintain, there will be more room for flexibility. But I have a very strong feeling that you will be so pleased with how you feel, and how amazingly quickly your cravings will have subsided, that you may not be as tempted to reach for the savory or sweet treats! I often tell people who admit to being sugar addicts that they will really, truly, and honestly lose their taste for it. Sometimes they look at me as if I'm bananas—but once they get going, they realize it's true!

- If you do overindulge, do what I do—and that means do not tell yourself you have no willpower and are a failure! Just add more cardio to your routine. Go for an extra hike, do one of the total-body workouts, or get outside and sweat any way you can. Then make sure that before your next meal you're drinking a lot of water or drinking one of my favorite teas. It will help curb your cravings and let you know if you're truly hungry or comfort-eating out of habit, boredom, or stress.

- I love my teas! They aren't just delicious—they're incredibly satisfying and therapeutic. I created them to fill in the gap during the day or after dinner when it's usually sweets-or-snack-craving time. Make your tea drinking a daily habit. That will soon become almost a ritual, and something uniquely wonderful you are doing for yourself. After lunch, which is when I tend to crave something sweet, I automatically head for my kitchen. I turn on the kettle and I make one of my teas. While it's brewing, I pick out a lovely cup. Then I enjoy every sip of it and get on with my day, satisfied, refreshed, and full of energy.

If you can follow these tips and stay focused on the shopping list on a week-to-week basis, you'll minimize your cravings, reduce the likelihood that you'll be buying and consuming processed foods, and be well on your way to maintaining the 5-6-7-8 plan!

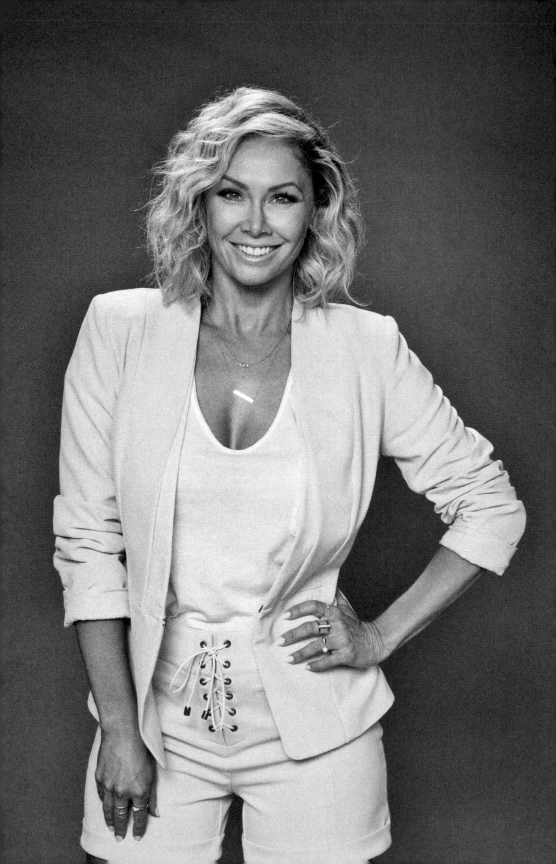

⑤

The 5-6-7-8 Recipes

I hope you will enjoy making these recipes as much as you'll enjoy eating them! You'll find lots more in chapter 11, too.

Teatime Recipes

Because drinking these teas is so important, I hope you'll make them a regular part of your day—and so they deserve to come first in this chapter!

As you know already, many people get hungry in the late afternoon or after dinner, and this is when the comfort eating can start. I got myself out of this habit by becoming a tea drinker. I'll admit to still being a coffee addict, but I've changed my ways so I just drink it black in the morning, and I've grown to love my wide assortment of teas. There are so many flavors to choose from, and when you drink them hot, they are very filling and satisfying. I tend to make them specifically when I'm vegging out on the couch while watching a movie . . . and thinking I might want to get something fattening to eat!

One item in my kitchen that I can't live without is my electric teakettle. It heats up the water quickly, and it shuts itself off when done, which is great if you forget that you put it on! I often make a pot of tea at night before bed, and then simply place the whole pot in the fridge overnight. Then I've got iced tea waiting for me in the morning.

How to Make a Proper Pot of Tea

I absolutely love my tea. I like to keep my teabags and loose-leaf teas in sealed jars in the kitchen to avoid spoiling their flavors. When you're making tea remember to use a clean teapot and warm it up by swirling some hot water in it before starting. Once I boil my water I like to pour it directly over my tea leaves or tea bags in the pot. It's rare I'll make just one cup of tea; I always use my teapot. I recommend one teaspoon of loose-leaf tea per person (or cup you plan to have) or one bag of tea for every two people. I like my tea on the weaker side so I let it brew for one and a half to two minutes, but you can certainly intensify its taste if you allow it to brew for three or more minutes. We've prepared four therapeutic teas—Detox Tea, Anti-inflammatory Tea, Sweet Comfort Tea, and Digestion Tea—as part of the 5-6-7-8 plan. I hope you enjoy them as much as I do!

Detox Tea

This tea is a delicious mixture of green tea, lemon, apple cider vinegar, and honey. It's my favorite tonic tea; I've found that's it's especially soothing when it's hot and especially refreshing when it's cold. If you are sensitive to caffeine, use decaf green tea or only drink this before three p.m.

Serves: 1

Ingredients
2 cups hot water

1 green tea bag

1/2 lemon, juiced

1 teaspoon honey

1 teaspoon apple cider vinegar

1. Bring water to a boil and steep tea bag for 3–4 minutes.
2. Add juice of lemon, honey, and apple cider vinegar and stir until blended.
3. Sip and enjoy!

Anti-inflammatory Tea

This tea features turmeric, a potent and pungent anti-inflammatory spice that is best known for its use in the cooking of India—it's what gives the vivid orange color to the super-nourishing dal, a dish of stewed lentils, and various curries.

Serves: 1

Ingredients

1 cup unsweetened light canned coconut milk

1 cup water

1 teaspoon turmeric

$1/4$ teaspoon ginger powder

1 teaspoon maple syrup

1. In a small saucepan, heat mixture for 3–5 minutes over medium heat while stirring occasionally.
2. Sip and enjoy!

Sweet Comfort Tea

This is the tea I find most satisfying when I'm craving chocolate or something sweet.

Serves: 1

Ingredients

1 cup unsweetened light canned coconut milk

$1/2$ cup water

1 tablespoon cacao powder

$1/2$ teaspoon cinnamon

Pinch of cayenne pepper (optional)

1. In a small saucepan, bring all ingredients to a boil while stirring occasionally.
2. Sip and enjoy!

Digestion Tea

The ginger and lemon aid in digestion, while the maple syrup adds a hint of sweetness and the cayenne a bit of snap.

Serves: 1

Ingredients

2 cups water

$1/4$-inch piece of fresh ginger, peeled and minced

1 teaspoon pure maple syrup

$1/2$ lemon, juiced

$1/2$ teaspoon cayenne pepper

1. Place all ingredients in a small saucepan and let simmer over low-medium heat for 7–10 minutes, stirring occasionally.
2. Sip and enjoy!

Katrina's Green Tea

My friend Katrina taught me how to make this super-refreshing tea. It's wonderful on a hot day.

Serves: 4

Ingredients

4 cups water

2 or 3 green tea bags

1 small cucumber, peeled and sliced

2 or 3 sprigs mint

2 or 3 drops mint chlorophyll (optional)

1. Bring water to a boil and steep tea bags for 3–4 minutes.
2. Place tea in refrigerator until it is chilled.
3. Add cucumber, mint, and mint chlorophyll (if desired). Stir gently.
4. Sip and enjoy!

Breakfast Recipes

I grew up eating a typical Australian breakfast. Either we had Weetabix, a whole-grain cereal that's not as sweet as most American cereals, with milk, or we had toast with Vegemite. I have yet to see Vegemite in an American pantry—it's definitely an Australian thing and an acquired taste that few people acquire if they don't grow up eating it! It's made from brewer's yeast, and it tastes quite salty, although the actual sodium content is low. I love it on whole-grain toast topped with a few slices of avocado. Not only is it filling but it satisfies any cravings I have for something salty.

Green Smoothie

I prefer my own smoothies to those already prepared as I can easily control the balance of green veggies to fruit. Have fun experimenting with your preferences, as each leafy green has its own distinctive taste.

Serves: 1

Ingredients

8 ounces nonfat plain Greek yogurt

1 kiwi, peeled

1 two-inch piece of cucumber, skinned

2 cups kale, chopped, or leafy greens of your choice

1 tablespoon honey

1 cup ice

1 cup water (more or less depending on your consistency preference)

1. Place all ingredients in a blender and puree until smooth.

Mocha Banana Nut Smoothie

Serves: 1

Ingredients

$1/2$ cup brewed coffee

$1/2$ cup unsweetened almond milk

$1/2$ banana

1 tablespoon cacao powder

2 tablespoons almond butter

1 cup ice

1. Place all ingredients in a blender and puree until smooth.

Spinach Goat Cheese Scramble

Serves: 1

Ingredients

2 whole eggs

Olive oil cooking spray

2 cups baby spinach

1 ounce goat cheese, or cheese of your choice

1 slice sprouted-grain bread, toasted

Salt and pepper, to taste

1. Whisk eggs in a small bowl.
2. Spray a skillet with olive oil spray and heat to medium heat.
3. Pour egg mixture into skillet and let cook for one minute.
4. Add spinach and cheese and stir frequently for 2–4 minutes or until eggs are set.
5. Season with salt and pepper and serve with toast.

Zucchini Goat Cheese Frittata

Frittatas are one of my favorite breakfast items. I'll often make one at night, store it in the refrigerator overnight, and then reheat it in the oven in the morning when I'm taking my shower and getting ready for the day.

Serves: 1

Ingredients

1 teaspoon olive oil

1 small zucchini, chopped

2 whole eggs

1 ounce goat cheese, or cheese of your choice

Salt and pepper, to taste

1 slice sprouted-grain bread, toasted

1. Place olive oil and zucchini in a skillet over medium heat and cook for about 2 minutes, or until zucchini starts to soften.
2. Whisk eggs together in a small bowl.
3. Pour egg mixture into skillet and stir slowly while reducing heat to medium-low.
4. Sprinkle with cheese, season with salt and pepper, and let cook until eggs set completely, about 2 more minutes.
5. Remove frittata with a spatula and serve with toast.

Cinnamon Greek Yogurt Parfait

Serves: 1

Ingredients

8 ounces nonfat plain Greek yogurt

1 cup fresh berries

2 tablespoons crushed almonds

1 tablespoon honey

$1/2$ teaspoon cinnamon

1. Place yogurt in a small bowl or mason jar and layer the berries and almonds.
2. Top with honey and cinnamon and serve.

Protein-Packed Pancake Recipes

Who doesn't love pancakes? For me, they've always been the ultimate comfort food. But as you know already, traditional pancakes are
often made with white flour, and they can be high in calories, especially if you add a lot of butter and syrup to them. So I've created twelve
protein-packed pancakes to meet the needs of the 5-6-7-8 Diet. The
pancake recipes here are made without white flour, and include ingredients like eggs, bananas, and Greek yogurt. They're a delicious and
lower-calorie alternative to your traditional pancakes. Enjoy!

NOTE: For all the pancake recipes, you can save calories by using a
coconut oil cooking spray when you're heating the pan instead of coconut oil. You can also reduce the amount of syrup, if desired, to ½ tablespoon, which will reduce the calories by about twenty-six. (Please
do not ever use table syrup, which is little more than calorie-dense and
non-nutritious high-fructose corn syrup and artificial flavors.) Sometimes you might be in the mood for pancakes that are more savory than
sweet; if so, you won't need any syrup at all!

Flourless Banana Pancakes

Serves: 1

Ingredients
1 banana
2 whole eggs
Pinch of baking powder
½ teaspoon cinnamon (optional)
1 teaspoon coconut oil
1 tablespoon pure maple syrup

1. Mash the banana in a small bowl.
2. Beat the eggs until smooth and add to banana. Add baking powder and cinnamon, if desired. Mix thoroughly.
3. Grease a nonstick frying pan or griddle well with the coconut oil. (An easy way
   to do this is to pour some onto a paper towel and wipe it on the pan; you don't

want too much oil when you make pancakes!) Heat the oil over medium heat for a minute or two.

4. Use a ladle to pour in some of the batter until the pancake is about the size of your palm. Repeat with the rest of the batter.

5. Cook until bubbles form on the surface and the bottom is browning nicely, about 30 seconds more.

6. Flip the pancakes and cook for about a minute more, until bottom is nicely browned.

7. Serve immediately with maple syrup.

Peaches 'n Cream Pancakes

Serves: 1

Ingredients

2 whole eggs

1 banana

Pinch of baking powder

Cinnamon, if desired

1 teaspoon coconut oil

$^{1}/_{2}$ peach, sliced

2 tablespoons plain nonfat Greek yogurt

1. Mix eggs, banana, baking powder, and cinnamon with a hand blender or in a blender.

2. Grease a nonstick frying pan or griddle well with the coconut oil or spray. Heat the oil over medium heat for a minute or two.

3. Use a ladle to pour in some of the batter until the pancake is about the size of your palm. Repeat with the rest of the batter.

4. Cook until bubbles form on the surface and the bottom is browning nicely, about 30 seconds more.

5. Flip the pancakes and cook for a minute more, until bottom is nicely browned.

6. Serve with sliced peaches and top with Greek yogurt and cinnamon, if desired.

Blueberry Oat Bran Pancakes

Serves: 1

Ingredients

1 whole egg

1 banana

1 tablespoon Greek yogurt

Pinch of salt (cinnamon, and vanilla, as desired)

$^1/_4$ cup oat bran

About 12 blueberries

1 teaspoon coconut oil

1 tablespoon pure maple syrup

1. Mix egg, banana, yogurt, and salt with a hand blender or in a blender.
2. Stir in oat bran and blueberries.
3. Grease a nonstick frying pan or griddle well with the coconut oil or spray. Heat the oil over medium heat for a minute or two.
4. Use a ladle to pour in some of the batter until the pancake is about the size of your palm. Repeat with the rest of the batter.
5. Cook until bubbles form on the surface and the bottom is browning nicely, about 30 seconds more.
6. Flip the pancakes and cook for about a minute more, until bottom is nicely browned.
7. Serve immediately with maple syrup.

Greek Yogurt Pancakes

Serves: 1

Ingredients

$^1/_4$ cup coconut flour

$^1/_4$ cup almond flour

Pinch of baking powder

6 ounces nonfat plain Greek yogurt

1 egg

$^1/_2$ teaspoon vanilla extract

1 teaspoon coconut oil

1 tablespoon pure maple syrup

1. Whisk together the dry ingredients, then add all of the wet ones except coconut oil and whisk until smooth.

2. Grease a nonstick frying pan or griddle well with the coconut oil or spray. Heat the oil over medium heat for a minute or two.
3. Use a ladle to pour in some of the batter until the pancake is about the size of your palm. Repeat with the rest of the batter.
4. Cook until bubbles form on the surface and the bottom is browning nicely, about 30 seconds more.
5. Flip the pancakes and cook for about a minute more, until bottom is nicely browned.
6. Serve immediately with maple syrup.

VARIATION: Add 12–15 fresh raspberries to the batter before ladling into the hot skillet.

Almond Butter or Peanut Butter Pancakes

Serves: 1

Ingredients

2 whole eggs

1 banana

Pinch of baking powder

1 tablespoon almond butter *or* peanut butter

1 teaspoon coconut oil or spray

1 tablespoon pure maple syrup

1. Mix eggs, banana, baking powder, and almond butter or peanut butter with a hand blender or in a blender.
2. Grease a nonstick frying pan or griddle well with the coconut oil or spray. Heat the oil over medium heat for a minute or two.
3. Use a ladle to pour in some of the batter until the pancake is about the size of your palm. Repeat with the rest of the batter.
4. Cook until bubbles form on the surface and the bottom is browning nicely, about 30 seconds more.
5. Flip the pancakes and cook for about a minute more, until bottom is nicely browned.
6. Serve immediately with maple syrup.

Fluffy Buckwheat Pancakes

Serves: 1

Ingredients

1 whole egg (yolks and whites separated)

1/4 cup plain nonfat Greek yogurt

1 teaspoon vanilla extract

1/4 cup buckwheat flour

1/2 tablespoon sugar

Pinch of fine sea salt

Pinch of baking powder

1 teaspoon coconut oil or spray

1 tablespoon pure maple syrup

1. Beat the egg yolk by hand until smooth; add Greek yogurt and vanilla extract.
2. In a separate bowl, mix together buckwheat flour, sugar, salt and baking power with a hand blender or in a blender
3. Pour the flour mixture into the egg mixture and mix to combine.
4. Whip egg whites until very stiff. Fold egg whites into batter gently, using a soft spatula.
5. Grease a nonstick frying pan or griddle well with the coconut oil or spray. Heat the oil over medium heat for a minute or two.
6. Use a ladle to pour in some of the batter until the pancake is about the size of your palm. Repeat with the rest of the batter.
7. Cook until bubbles form on the surface and the bottom is browning nicely, about 30 seconds more.
8. Flip the pancakes and cook for about a minute more, until bottom is nicely browned.
9. Serve immediately with maple syrup.

Vanilla Protein Pancakes

Serves: 1

Ingredients

2 whole eggs

1 banana

Pinch of baking powder

1/2 teaspoon cinnamon

2 tablespoons vanilla protein powder

1 teaspoon coconut oil or spray

1 tablespoon pure maple syrup

1. Mix eggs, banana, baking powder, cinnamon, and protein powder with a hand blender or in a blender.

2. Grease a nonstick frying pan or griddle well with the coconut oil or spray. Heat the oil over medium heat for a minute or two.
3. Use a ladle to pour in some of the batter until the pancake is about the size of your palm. Repeat with the rest of the batter.
4. Cook until bubbles form on the surface and the bottom is browning nicely, about 30 seconds more.
5. Flip the pancakes and cook for about a minute more, until bottom is nicely browned.
6. Serve immediately with maple syrup.

Chocolate Protein Pancakes

Serves: 1

Ingredients

2 whole eggs

1 banana

Pinch of baking powder

$1/2$ teaspoon cinnamon

2 tablespoons chocolate protein powder

1 teaspoon coconut oil or spray

1. Mix eggs, banana, baking powder, cinnamon, and protein powder with a hand blender or in a blender.
2. Grease a nonstick frying pan or griddle well with the coconut oil or spray. Heat the oil over medium heat for a minute or two.
3. Use a ladle to pour in some of the batter until the pancake is about the size of your palm. Repeat with the rest of the batter.
4. Cook until bubbles form on the surface and the bottom is browning nicely, about 30 seconds more.
5. Flip the pancakes and cook for about a minute more, until bottom is nicely browned.

Coconut Pancakes

Serves: 1

Ingredients

2 whole eggs

1 banana

Pinch of baking powder

1 tablespoon unsweetened shredded coconut

1 teaspoon coconut oil or spray

1 tablespoon pure maple syrup

1. Mix eggs, banana, baking powder, and shredded coconut with a hand blender or in a blender.
2. Grease a nonstick frying pan or griddle well with the coconut oil or spray. Heat the oil over medium heat for a minute or two.
3. Use a ladle to pour in some of the batter until the pancake is about the size of your palm. Repeat with the rest of the batter.
4. Cook until bubbles form on the surface and the bottom is browning nicely, about 30 seconds more.
5. Flip the pancakes and cook for about a minute more, until bottom is nicely browned.
6. Serve immediately with maple syrup.

Almond Paleo Pancakes

Serves: 3

Ingredients

1 cup almond flour	1 egg
1 teaspoon coconut flour	1 tablespoon honey
Pinch of baking soda	1 tablespoon coconut oil or spray
Pinch of kosher salt	$1/2$ cup almond milk

1. Whisk together the dry ingredients, then add all of wet ones except coconut oil and whisk until smooth.
2. Grease a nonstick frying pan or griddle well with the coconut oil or spray. Heat the oil over medium heat for a minute or two.

3. Use a ladle to pour in some of the batter until the pancake is about the size of your palm. Repeat with the rest of the batter.
4. Cook until bubbles form on the surface and the bottom is browning nicely, about 30 seconds more.
5. Flip the pancakes and cook for about a minute more, until bottom is nicely browned

Apple Cinnamon Oatmeal Pancakes

Serves: 2

Ingredients

1 whole egg

$1/2$ cup oatmeal

$1/2$ cup skim milk

Pinch of cinnamon

1 teaspoon coconut oil or spray

$1/2$ apple, cored and chopped

3 walnuts, crushed

1 tablespoon pure maple syrup

1. Mix eggs, oatmeal, milk, and cinnamon with a hand blender or in a blender.
2. Grease a nonstick frying pan or griddle well with the coconut oil or spray. Heat the oil over medium heat for a minute or two, then add apples.
3. Let apples cook for about 3 minutes, stirring occasionally, then remove them from the skillet and place on a plate.
4. Use a ladle to pour in some of the batter until the pancake is about the size of your palm. Repeat with the rest of the batter.
5. Cook until bubbles form on the surface and the bottom is browning nicely, about 30 seconds more.
6. Flip the pancakes and cook for about a minute more, until bottom is nicely browned.
7. Serve immediately, topped with cooked apples, and top with cinnamon, walnuts, and maple syrup.

Lemon Poppy Seed Pancakes

Serves: 1

Ingredients

1/4 cup coconut flour

1/4 cup almond flour

Pinch of baking powder

1 teaspoon lemon zest

1 teaspoon poppy seeds or chia seeds

6 ounces nonfat plain Greek yogurt
   or nonfat ricotta

1 egg

1/2 teaspoon vanilla extract

1 teaspoon coconut oil

1/2 tablespoon pure maple syrup

1. Whisk together the dry ingredients, then add all of wet ones except coconut oil and maple syrup and whisk until smooth.
2. Grease a nonstick frying pan or griddle well with the coconut oil or spray. Heat the oil over medium heat for a minute or two.
3. Use a ladle to pour in some of the batter until the pancake is about the size of your palm. Repeat with the rest of the batter.
4. Cook until bubbles form on the surface and the bottom is browning nicely, about 30 seconds more.
5. Flip the pancakes and cook for about a minute more, until bottom is nicely browned.
5. Serve immediately with maple syrup.

Lunch Recipes

When I'm dancing, I tend to eat a fairly light lunch, as it's hard to spend an afternoon rehearsing on a full stomach. When I'm not dancing, however, I enjoy more food at lunchtime, so dig in! In fact, I prefer to eat a larger lunch and lighter dinner whenever possible. If you're planning to cook for a friend or your family, these recipes can easily be doubled or tripled.

Quinoa Bowl with Roasted Vegetables

Serves: 1

Ingredients

³/₄ cup quinoa, cooked

1 small zucchini, chopped

¹/₂ carrot, chopped

1 small yellow squash, chopped

¹/₄ small red onion, chopped

1 tablespoon coconut oil

Sea salt, to taste

1 teaspoon fresh rosemary

1 tablespoon fresh lemon juice

1. Preheat oven to 400 degrees.
2. Cook quinoa according to directions on the package.
3. Place veggies on a roasting tray, drizzle with oil (coconut oil must be in liquid form; if yours has solidified, which coconut oil can do if the kitchen isn't particularly warm, heat it for about 20–30 seconds in the microwave, or until it melts), and season with salt and herbs.
4. Roast in the oven until tender, about 15 minutes.
5. Toss quinoa together with veggies and sprinkle fresh lemon juice on top.

Arugula, Olive, and Grilled Chicken Salad

Serves: 1

Ingredients

cooking spray

4 ounces boneless chicken breast

2 cups arugula

1 medium carrot, peeled and chopped

6 Kalamata olives, halved and pitted

1 ounce roasted pumpkin seeds

1 teaspoon olive oil

$^1/_2$ lemon, juiced

Salt and pepper

1. Preheat grill or grill pan to medium heat, and spray the grill or the pan with cooking spray.
2. Grill chicken for 6–7 minutes on each side, or until cooked through or the chicken reaches your desired temperature.
3. Assemble arugula and peeled carrot on a plate and top with chicken, olives, pumpkin seeds, olive oil, and lemon juice. Season with salt and pepper to taste.

Salmon Niçoise Salad

Serves: 1

Ingredients

3 ounces salmon (canned or fresh)

1 egg, hard-boiled

2 cups salad greens

$^1/_4$ small red onion, thinly sliced

$^1/_2$ cup green beans, steamed

2 tablespoons Kalamata olives, chopped

1 tablespoon capers

1 teaspoon olive oil

$^1/_2$ lemon, juiced

Salt and pepper

1. If using fresh salmon, spray skillet with olive oil spray, and place salmon in skillet over medium heat. If using canned salmon, place in salad bowl.
2. Cook salmon until slightly browned and flaky, about five minutes each side.
3. Assemble all ingredients except olive oil, lemon juice, and salt and pepper in a salad bowl.
4. Dress with olive oil and squeezed lemon juice, and season with salt and pepper to taste.

Black Bean Avocado Salad

Serves: 1

Ingredients

1/2 cup cooked brown rice

2 cups salad greens

1/2 cup black beans, cooked or canned

1/4 avocado, cubed

1/4 small onion, chopped (optional)

1 tablespoon chopped cilantro

1 teaspoon olive oil

1/2 lime, juiced

Salt and pepper

Hot sauce or salsa to taste

1. Layer the brown rice, salad greens, and beans.
2. Top with avocado, onion, and cilantro.
3. Dress with olive oil, lime, salt, pepper, and hot sauce to taste.

Pasta, Peas, and Pesto

Serves: 1

Ingredients

1 cup fusilli or farfalle pasta

1 tablespoon pesto

1/2 cup baby tomatoes, halved

1 cup frozen peas, thawed

Salt and pepper

1. Cook pasta according to package instructions.
2. Add cooked pasta, pesto, tomatoes, and peas to a bowl and toss.
3. Season with salt and pepper.

Open-faced SALT
(Salmon, Avocado, Lettuce, Tomato) Sandwich

Serves: 1

Ingredients

Olive oil spray

4 ounces salmon

1/4 avocado, mashed

1 slice sprouted-grain bread

2 lettuce leaves (Romaine lettuce
would be best)

2 slices tomato

Salt and pepper

1. Spray skillet with olive oil spray, and place salmon in it over medium heat.
2. Cook salmon until slightly browned and flaky, about 5 minutes each side.
3. Spread avocado on bread, and add lettuce and tomato.
4. Top with salmon, and season with salt and pepper to taste.

Basic Vinaigrette

This should become one of your go-to weapons in the 5-6-7-8 Diet Plan arsenal! You can use plain oil and vinegar to taste, of course, but a homemade vinaigrette takes about a minute to make, and the flavor is so far superior to what comes out of a salad-dressing bottle that you'll wonder why you ever used them. Using the same proportions, try experimenting with different oils, spices, and mustards as each will give the vinaigrette a different flavor. For a mustard vinaigrette, add one teaspoon Dijon mustard. For a lemon or orange vinaigrette, replace the vinegar with lemon or orange juice. For a creamy vinaigrette, add one or two tablespoons of plain Greek yogurt. You can also whip this up in the morning or when you first start cooking and let it stand to improve the flavor. Just whisk it a bit with a fork before you pour it on your salad.

Serves: 2

Ingredients

3 tablespoons oil, preferably olive, walnut, or sesame

2 tablespoons vinegar, preferably white wine or apple cider

Salt and pepper

1. Whisk the oil and vinegar together until smooth.
2. Season with salt and pepper to taste.

Dinner Recipes

These dinner recipes are some of my favorite things to serve at home, whether I'm on my own or entertaining guests. You'll notice that you don't feel as if you're "going without" when you're enjoying them. These delicious meals provide a healthy balance of protein, veggies, and complex carbs to help you stay on track with the 5-6-7-8 plan.

Turkey Burger with Spicy Sweet Potato "Fries"

Serves: 1

Ingredients for Burger

1 turkey burger patty

2 slices tomato

2 big lettuce leaves

2 slices pickle

Hot sauce or mustard to taste

Ingredients for Sweet Potato Fries

1 medium sweet potato, cut into
    wedges

1 teaspoon coconut oil (melted)

Cumin, a few dashes

Cayenne, a few dashes

Salt, a few dashes

For Burger

1. Grill or cook burger in a lightly sprayed pan until cooked to your preferred doneness.
2. Stack burger ingredients on lettuce and top with second lettuce leaf.

For Sweet Potato Fries

1. Preheat oven to 400 degrees.
2. In a small bowl, place all ingredients and mix until potatoes are evenly coated with oil and spices to taste.
3. Roast for about 30 minutes, turning once.

Steak Plate with Spinach and Grilled Mushrooms

Serves: 1

Ingredients

4 ounces flank steak

Salt and pepper, to taste

cooking spray

2 portobello mushrooms, divided

2 teaspoons balsamic vinegar

2 cups baby spinach

1 tablespoon olive oil

1 tablespoon grated
  Parmesan cheese

1. Season steak on both sides with salt and pepper, if desired.
2. Using a medium nonstick skillet or grill pan, spray pan with cooking spray and cook steak over medium-high heat for 8 minutes on each side, or until it reaches desired degree of doneness.
3. While the steak is cooking, season mushroom caps with 1 teaspoon vinegar, salt, and pepper, and add to the grill or pan.
4. Cook the mushrooms for 10 minutes.
5. Remove steak from heat and place it on a cutting board to slice diagonally.
6. Remove mushrooms when cooked, and slice on top of spinach.
7. Dress salad with olive oil and remaining teaspoon of vinegar. Place sliced steak on top of salad and top with Parmesan cheese.

Beets, Feta, and Grilled Chicken Salad

Serves: 1

Ingredients

4 ounces chicken breast

2 boiled beets, quartered

2 cups salad greens

2 ounces feta cheese, cubed

$^1/_2$ tablespoon olive oil

1 tablespoon balsamic vinegar

Salt and pepper

1. Grill or bake chicken breast.
2. Assemble all ingredients on a plate, and dress with olive oil, vinegar, salt, and pepper to taste.

Ginger Shrimp and Broccoli Stir-fry

Serves: 1

Ingredients

$^1/_2$ cup brown rice

1 teaspoon coconut oil

$^1/_4$ onion, sliced

1 clove garlic, minced

1 teaspoon fresh ginger, minced
    or grated

4 ounces shrimp, peeled and deveined

2 cups broccoli florets

1 teaspoon tamari or soy sauce

4 tablespoons stock (can be veggie, chicken, or beef; preferably
    homemade)

1. Cook rice according to package instructions.
2. Heat a skillet with coconut oil over medium-high heat.
3. Add onions, garlic, and ginger, and cook until onions become translucent, about 2–3 minutes.
4. Add shrimp and cook for about 1 minute on each side, until the shrimp are seared.
5. Lower heat to medium; add broccoli florets, tamari or soy sauce, and stock; and cover.
6. Let cook for another 3–4 minutes or until shrimp are completely cooked through and opaque.
7. Serve over brown rice.

Spinach, Apple, Quinoa, and Goat Cheese Salad

If you're not crazy about goat cheese, feel free to substitute any other cheese that you like or remove it altogether.

Serves: 1

Ingredients

$1/2$ green or Granny Smith apple, cored and diced

1 tablespoon lemon juice

2 cups baby spinach

1 tablespoon virgin olive oil

$1/2$ tablespoon apple cider vinegar

$1/2$ teaspoon honey

Salt and pepper, to taste

$1/4$ cup crumbled goat cheese

$1/2$ cup quinoa, cooked

$1/8$ cup chopped walnuts

1. Toss apple with lemon juice.
2. Place spinach in a salad bowl.
3. Whisk together olive oil, vinegar, honey, and salt and pepper to taste.
4. Pour dressing over spinach and top with apples, cheese, quinoa, and walnuts.

Florence Henderson's Savory Coconut Rice

Florence is a dear friend and fabulous cook. I'd take a lesson from her any day!

Serves: 2

Ingredients

2 cups water

$1/2$ tablespoon butter or olive oil

Salt, a few dashes

1 cup brown rice

$1/4$ cup unsweetened flaked coconut

$1/4$ cup chopped toasted nuts (cashews, almonds, hazelnuts)

1. Bring water, butter or olive oil, salt, and rice to a boil in a saucepan.
2. Reduce heat to low, cover, and simmer for about 20 minutes, or until rice is cooked and fluffy.
3. Remove from heat and add coconut and nuts. Mix well. Serve immediately.

Steamed Salmon and Broccoli Over Cauliflower Mash

Serves: 1

Ingredients for Salmon and Broccoli

4 ounces salmon

1 cup broccoli florets

1–2 tablespoons Dijon mustard

Salt and pepper

2 tablespoons crushed hazelnuts

Ingredients for Cauliflower Mash

$^1/_4$ medium cauliflower head

⅛ cup unsweetened almond milk

Salt and pepper, to taste

1 teaspoon fresh chives

Garlic powder, to taste

Directions for Salmon and Broccoli

1. Preheat oven to 400 degrees.
2. Place salmon and broccoli together in a tinfoil pouch, and cover with Dijon mustard.
3. Flavor with a touch of salt and some black pepper, and add crushed hazelnuts.
4. Seal the pouch, and bake for about 20 minutes or until the salmon flakes with a fork.

Directions for Cauliflower Mash

1. Steam cauliflower and place in a food processor or blender.
2. Add rest of ingredients and blend until smooth.
3. Spread cauliflower mash on the plate, and top with salmon and broccoli.

Snack Recipes

These are all super easy and super filling!

Greek Yogurt and Berries

Serves: 1

Ingredients

1 cup plain low-fat Greek yogurt

1 cup berries (your choice)

1 teaspoon honey

1. Layer yogurt and berries.
2. Top with honey and enjoy.

Snap Peas and Hummus

Serves: 1

Ingredients

2 cups snap peas

1/4 cup hummus

1. Cut snap peas into 1/4-inch pieces.
2. Dip into hummus and enjoy.

Edamame, Lemon, and Salt

Serves: 1

Ingredients

Salt, a few pinches

Fresh lemon juice, a few squeezes

3/4 cup shelled, cooked edamame

Add salt and lemon juice to edamame, and enjoy.

Cinnamon Chia Pudding

Serves: 1

Ingredients

1 cup unsweetened almond milk

1/4 cup chia seeds

1 tablespoon maple syrup

1/2 teaspoon cinnamon

1. Mix almond milk, chia seeds, maple syrup, and cinnamon together in a small bowl or mason jar.
2. Let sit overnight in the refrigerator so the chia seeds gelatinize.
3. Stir well and enjoy.

DIY Trail Mix

Serves: 1

Ingredients

$^1/_2$ ounce raw almonds

$^1/_4$ ounce dried cranberries

$^1/_2$ ounce pumpkin seeds

Mix all ingredients together and enjoy.

Dark Chocolate Almond Butter Balls

Serves: 1

Ingredients

1 tablespoon almond butter

2 tablespoons rolled oats

1 tablespoon dark chocolate chips

1. Mix all ingredients together and form 1-inch balls.
2. Refrigerate the balls for at least 10 minutes.
3. Serve and enjoy.

Apple with Almond Butter

Serves: 1

Ingredients

1 small apple, cored and sliced

1 tablespoon almond butter

Spread almond butter on the apple slices, and enjoy.

Egg on a Brown Rice Cake

Serves: 1

Ingredients

1 brown rice cake

1 egg, hard-boiled and sliced

Top the rice cake with the egg, and enjoy.

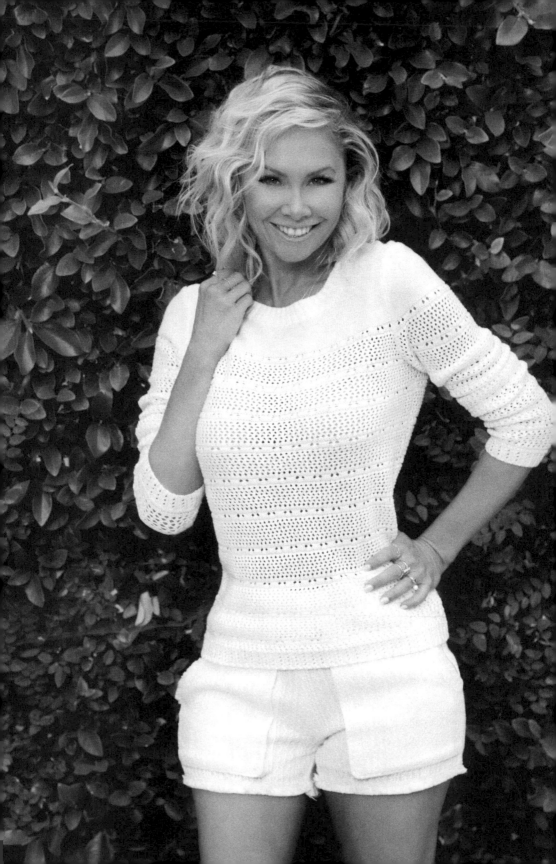

Part III

The 5-6-7-8 Workouts

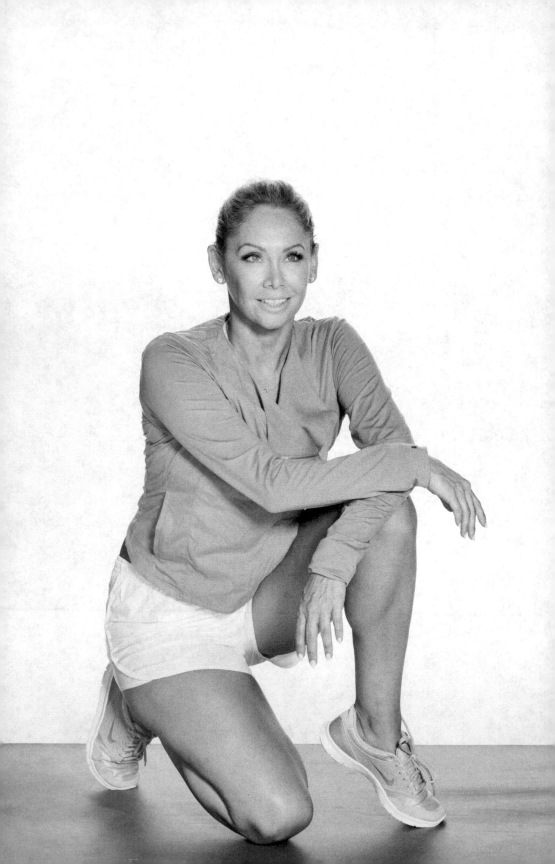

6

My Fitness Philosophy

I've been dancing nearly my entire life and have been blessed with many nurturing and encouraging teachers. I've also been blessed with equally wonderful colleagues and friends who've helped me be the best possible performer. I've consolidated some of their tips for you here to help you stay motivated throughout your health and fitness journey.

Over the years, I've developed my own philosophy about the most effective workouts to help me achieve and maintain a lean, sculpted dancer's body. I hope these lessons and thoughts will help guide you and keep you motivated on your way to a healthy, beautiful, vibrant body.

Be Prepared

Appearing on *Dancing with the Stars* is very challenging for non-dancers. It's so completely outside of their comfort zone that I needed to choreograph a dance, rehearse it, maximize the results, and steady the nerves of my partners in a very short time. As a pro you want to help your partner achieve their personal best, and so you need to be mentally and emotionally prepared to support them.

At the start of every season, all the professional dancers request the songs they want to use that match the tempo of the dances we'll be doing. Sometimes you get what you want; sometimes you don't—and sometimes you only get the music the night before that week's rehearsals start. When that happened, I'd be up all night working out the steps so I'd have a good idea of what to do in the morning. Trust me, it's very hard to choreograph a dance without music!

I like to be prepared for when I walk into the studio—to go in there with a clear concept and creative idea of what I want to do. I don't like to choreograph on the spot, as I find it confuses my partners. I like to start from the beginning, move on to the middle, and then finish with the end. That's how I choreograph each dance and how I like to teach it, as this way my partners can build on each sequence and it's easier for them to remember. Then, during rehearsals, once my partners have gotten the basic steps down, we spend the rest of the week refining the dances till they're ready to perform.

My partners (and the audience!) don't know how much work goes into the process before the rehearsals even begin—and, actually, they don't need to know, either! That's part of my job. But it's important for you to know, because being prepared makes exercising so much more productive and satisfying. And fun!

Keep this in mind as you prepare to do your own exercising, because an integral part of the 5-6-7-8 philosophy is that you prepare diligently. Get your doctor's approval (especially if you have any health issues), plan when you're going to do your work out, set aside the time, and keep to the workout calendar. These plans are meant to be fun, but, like for any skill, they will require commitment from you to get the results you want.

Everyone Worries that They'll Mess Up

Nervous about exercising or learning new skills? Don't worry! Even pros like me get jitters. On my first season with *Dancing with the Stars* in

America, my partner was Jerry Springer. I felt so much pressure to have him do well—as I do with all my partners. Especially because you know the celebrities are getting judged, but it's what *you're* doing that they're being judged on. I was terrified during my first performance with Jerry. I wanted to make sure he looked good, and luckily it couldn't have gone better. America fell in love with this kindhearted man and I was so relieved afterward. He was, too!

The celebrities on the show are super nervous at first, particularly if they have little or no dance experience. When I first met my partners, I asked about their dance experience, and then I asked if they did yoga (which would help with flexibility and breathing) or if they were active (which would help with muscle strength and coordination). Then I needed to see how they moved, naturally, so I asked them to show me how they'd dance around the house if music was playing, or how they'd dance at a nightclub. Some of my partners looked at me with panic in their eyes when I asked that and said, "Oh no, I would never do that!" That was when I knew I had to make them feel extra-confident about dancing. It's really satisfying to see people who never considered themselves "musical" learn how to move in tempo. And trust me, if someone who is terrified about dancing in public can do it live on national television, you can learn how to do all the exercises in this book in the comfort of your own home! I promise!

Set an Intention Before You Start to Move

Setting an intention is an extremely easy and valuable technique for putting yourself in the right mental space for exercise. I always take the time to do that before I begin a rehearsal or a workout. I give myself a mental checklist, and I feel like that sets up my brain to tell my body what to do. Acknowledging my goals makes them easier to envision, and to accomplish.

When I'm teaching my celebrities, I have the whole session planned out. I set out the tasks we have to hit and I want to make sure I get the first four counts of eight done before we take a break. We'll keep at it until our intention becomes reality. Earning the break is very satisfying!

Start at the Very Beginning

My friends like to tease me about what a bossy little girl I used to be, because I was always asking them to put on a show with me at school, and I used to make them rehearse with me during lunch when all they wanted to do was sit down and eat their sandwiches! After school, my dance friends would come back to my house and I'd say, yet again, "Let's put on a show!" I was always the director/choreographer. We'd perform our routines for their parents when they came to pick my friends up later. Sometimes I'd beg my brother to be in my "shows," too, which he hated. So I've always loved to teach and make up steps.

Still, it's taken me many years to become a confident teacher and know that I can pass along the skills that I've been taught so well. I learned how to choreograph by picking up little bits and pieces from the teachers who influenced me over the years. I took thousands and thousands of classes and worked really hard. I was fortunate to have learned from the best.

One of the best is Jason Gilkison, a world-champion ballroom dancer and the director and choreographer of *Burn the Floor*. He's been my mentor, and he taught me how to format and structure choreography, which is a very particular skill. Even if it doesn't appear so to an audience, all dances have a beginning, a middle, and an end. When you're creating a dance, it has to be broken down into each individual step, and then each step is built upon until it's complete. You need to start at the very beginning with the very first step before you can move on. Isn't that always the way? In dance, in exercise—and in everything else in life!

I've taught students of all different skill levels, but one of my most valuable teaching moments came as a result of teaching children with Down syndrome. These kids were such a joy to be around. After teaching that incredible group I've learned to make things a little more simple. When I first started teaching classes, I assumed that my students not only knew how to do basic moves but had the muscle strength to perform them. I quickly learned not to make any assumptions like that, especially when I saw the newbies struggling. Instead, I switched to the very simplest of basics. My students were thrilled when they completed easy dance or exercise sequences. That gave them an instant burst of confidence that they could master more complicated steps and moves. I mention this now, because all the workouts in this book have been designed for you to follow that approach. You'll first learn some target-area-specific workouts, then combine various exercises into a total-body fitness routine. Some movements may be challenging for you at first, but the breakdowns of each step as well as the photos should help you quickly master each routine.

Over the years, I've also become better at gauging the personalities of my students and partners, and adjusting my teaching accordingly. I had one celebrity on *Dancing with the Stars* who said to me right off the bat, "I just want to let you know that I've got ADD, I'm dyslexic, and I've got really terrible stage fright, okay?" I was taken aback, but instead of showing my surprise I thanked them and we got to work. This person was trying so hard yet was unable to even look in the mirror at first, because they would get confused between right and left. Instead of calling out right or left, which I normally do, I would tap their leg instead. The lesson for me was to be patient, to start at the very beginning every single time, to repeat the steps over and over and over again. It was an incredible learning experience and I had to hold on to the confidence that eventually everything would come together. This celebrity worked so hard and really did learn how to overcome both the learning issues and the stage fright. That was an amazing journey for us both and I'm so proud of how far my partner came.

Make Exercise Part of Your Lifestyle.

Some of the celebrities I worked with were extremely busy at their jobs and didn't have much time to rehearse. With Jerry Springer, we'd do no more than three hours a day (and I was worried, because, as you know, it was my very first season in America and I wanted to do my best!). Some days when he was taping his show we couldn't rehearse at all. Joey Fatone loved to rehearse and we'd often do eight hours a day. And Donny Osmond—wow! He was performing in Las Vegas when he was competing on the show. We would rehearse from ten a.m. to four p.m.

every single day without fail, and then he'd head off to the theater to perform with his sister, Marie! The man had so much energy, as well as talent and charisma. His work ethic and commitment were second to none, and he made dance part of his daily routine.

The bottom line is, when you make exercising a priority, it becomes just another part of your day and your lifestyle. Soon, you won't remember what it was like when you didn't exercise! You'll be amazed at how much more energy you have. And once you start to see results, you'll become even more motivated to keep going.

Donny Osmond on Fitness, Motivation, and Winning the Mirror Ball

I started performing at the age of five. Tap was my first style of dance. Actually my mom put me in a ballet class before that, but I'd rather forget about that since I was required to wear a leotard. Then over the years, I learned several other styles of dance. But I had never taken a ballroom dance class until I met Kym.

I had been working in Vegas for about a year and a half before competing on *Dancing with the Stars*. There is a lot of dancing in that show, but despite all of those cardio workouts onstage, I would still go to the gym three times a week and work on weight lifting to keep my muscle tone. I've had a pretty strict regimen for years. When I performed *Joseph and the Amazing Technicolor Dreamcoat*, I had great motivation to work out five times a week—because when all you wear onstage is a loincloth, you practically live at the gym!

So I thought I was in pretty good shape before *Dancing with the Stars*, but I had no idea how out of shape I was until Kym showed up and made me do these crazy dance moves. Especially as I had to do better than third place. That's how far Marie made it. I would never have lived it down if I didn't do better than third place. (If you recall, she got a lot of press after she fainted. But . . . I got the trophy. And I remind her of that every time I perform with her. Thank you, Kym!)

After my first rehearsal, there were muscles so sore in places I never even knew I had. I still have nightmares about going to the rehearsal hall at the Fern Adair Conservatory of the Arts in Las Vegas, let alone stepping onto the dance floor knowing millions of people are going to be judging a dance that I've had just about four days to learn. Oh, yeah. Don't forget about Len Goodman. That would give anyone anxiety! There's always that bit of doubt that pops into your mind, but Kym would always be positive and say, "You're ready. Now go have fun."

To this day, I have no idea where my energy came from. I really don't think I slept for about ten weeks. But what's really interesting is that after about week seven, if you're still in the competition, that Mirror Ball trophy is in sight, and I knew there just might be a chance I could get it despite bruised ribs, a broken toe, and shattered nerves. You just dream of holding that trophy and calling it yours. I joke about how tough Kym was, but to be honest with you, she is one of the nicest people I know. It's strange how she can work you to death but at the same time you like her for it because she has the sweetest personality.

When I went out there for our first dance, I was scared to death. I've been performing onstage for over fifty years, but that *Dancing with the Stars* stage was daunting. But it was probably one of the most exciting times of my career.

Still, during week seven, Kym and I had three different dances to do on the show. I had just finished the first dance and completely messed it up. The judges were really hard on me. I had really disappointed Kym as well. We were at the bottom of the leaderboard. So I'm backstage walking down the hall with my head down waiting for our turn to do our second dance, and I'm beating myself up for messing up that first dance. The next thing I know, my son Don had snuck backstage and grabbed me by my jacket collar. He backed me up against the wall and said, "Now, you get back out there and be the professional that I know you are, and that you know you are." That was the turning point for me. Kym and I climbed that leaderboard every week thereafter.

The night before the final performance, we were in the rehearsal hall. It was about eleven thirty p.m. We needed to be at the studio at six a.m. We had been rehearsing all day. I was so tired, lying there on the floor. I swear my feet were bleeding. I just couldn't get up. Kym demanded to go through the routine one more time. I said, "I just can't do it." Then she said something to me I'll never forget. It was simple but so succinct and to the point. And with her words, I found a strength in me I thought I didn't have. She said, "Do you want to win or not?" We won!

I only started to feel comfortable and think of myself as a dancer when Tom Bergeron handed me the trophy. And of course, flying on the private jet all night to New York and appearing on *Good Morning America* the following morning with Kym. We were dead tired but the crowd was so enthusiastic that it didn't matter. But I guess the best time that I realized Kym and I had just won the ultimate dance competition was about two weeks after the win. There was a little ten-year-old boy who came to see me perform in Vegas. After the show, during the meet-and-greet, he walked up to me, shook my hand, and said, "Mr. Osmond, I didn't know you could sing, too."

Since I did the show, I've been really aware of my posture, and I've changed my workout regimen. I've learned from Kym and from so many other personal trainers that it's all about core strength and not necessarily muscle mass. Yes, it's nice to have a great-looking physique, but that is secondary to core strength. My dancing continues with all of the shows that I do. After winning *Dancing with the Stars*, people expect me to keep my dancing skills in shape.

Everyone Learns How to Exercise in a Different Way

When learning a new skill, everyone is different.

With dance steps or exercises, some people like more repetition. Some of my partners like to break it down and write every little step in a notebook (they're verbal learners). I've found that most people are visual learners—they need to see the steps, over and over. Some visual learners ask me to break it down doing their steps, just by myself, which helps them envision how they'll be doing it.

For visual learners, sometimes during rehearsals I'd go to the next studio and grab one of the male pro dancers and ask them to do the steps with me. That way my partners could see the entire dance, with someone else doing their part, and that would be the catalyst they needed to perfect the routine.

One of my trade secrets is that I always made sure to film my rehearsals on an iPad so we could have an instant playback of the routine. I could be telling my partners over and over again what to do and how to hold their arms to make a turn, but only when they saw themselves, with me, did the information stick.

You likely already know what kind of learner you are. If you're a visual learner, the photos in this book will help you understand how you should position your body for the optimal results. You can also check out 5-6-7-8 Fitness (officialkymjohnson.com/5678-fitness), watch other DVDs, or stream exercise tips online to help you grasp the movements. If you're an aural learner, read the instructions over and over, and repeat them aloud. If you're a verbal learner, read the instructions first until you've got them clear in your head. This will make the process a lot smoother, and you'll memorize the exercises more quickly.

Don't Be Afraid to Look at Yourself— Proper Form Is Crucial

What's the first thing you see when you walk into a dance studio? Wall-to-wall mirrors. That's because dancers know they must constantly watch themselves to see what they're doing. We have to ensure that our alignment is correct and that we are performing the way the choreographer intended. I've had some of my celebrity partners say, "I don't want to look in the mirror and see what I'm doing. I hate seeing myself. I look terrible." But I know they have to start looking . . . so I'll ease them into it by having them start with their back to the mirrors. After a while I turn them around and when they end up seeing what they're doing they're usually blown away. The mirror really helps, because more often than not they say, "Wow, I'm not as bad as I thought I was!" or " It doesn't look as strange as it feels!"

It's not narcissistic to look at yourself when you're working out. On the contrary—it is a very necessary part of exercising. You need to be sure you are performing the moves correctly, and the only way to do that is to look. If you're doing things wrong, you're not going to get the results you want, and you might even injure yourself. Sometimes I think I'm doing a move perfectly, and then I look in the mirror and I realize I am completely off on one side, or my arms are not where I thought they were. Even experienced professionals can feel one thing—and be certain it's right—and then see the moves and realize they were wrong!

So my recommendation is that you try to do the routines in this book in front of a mirror if at all possible—even if only to familiarize yourself with the new movements you'll be learning. Otherwise, pay attention to the cues and instructions as you follow along with the routines.

Be Realistic

Even though I am a professional dancer and have been taking lessons for almost my entire life, that doesn't mean I don't have insecurities about my body. I have to work hard to stay in shape, especially as I'm getting older. We all have problem areas and flabby bits that haunt us, don't we!

So if you are new to exercise it's important you realize this will be a process. I always tell my friends who've had babies and are fretting about their baby weight afterward that it took nine months for the little miracle to grow inside their body, and they should expect at least nine months for the weight to come off. That's being realistic. And when you are, you can start to . . .

Love Your Body!

If you don't love your body, you won't be able to look in the mirror. So it's time to give yourself a fierce hug and love your body. It's the only one you have.

Instead of saying, "Oh, I can't stand to look at my belly," say, "Look at me doing these lunges. I am getting stronger every day."

No matter what size or shape you're in now, your body belongs to you. Embrace it. Love it. Be proud of it. And look at it fully in the mirror and acknowledge that you will be doing everything possible to make this wonderful body of yours as strong and healthy as it can be.

Your Body Is Unique to You—Don't Compare It to Anyone Else's

During the *Dancing with the Stars* rehearsals, we're all in one building. I would tell my celebrities not to start watching or comparing themselves to the other celebrities or dancers. That it's their journey to go on, as cheesy as that may sound.

So I'd give them my pep talk: "You can't compare yourself to anyone else because you'll psych yourself out," I'd tell them, "and you may have something that's great in a completely different way. So please don't start being in competition with the others. It's only about you; you're competing with yourself. That's all you can worry about. You can't worry about the others or what they're doing or what song they have. Just focus on what you can do and what you're best at."

Soon enough, the message would sink in!

I grew up competing in ballroom dancing against stunningly beautiful women. I had to learn at an early age to try to stop comparing myself to them and to anyone else. It can be very difficult—and yes, it's human nature to judge yourself against others. I know how hard it is not to do that. And it might be so frustrating when your best friend is lucky enough to have the kind of metabolism where she can pretty much eat what she wants and not gain a lot of weight. It's so unfair, right? But comparing yourself to her won't do anything except make you feel bad.

The only person that really counts is you.

And because your body is unique, you should realize that . . .

Everyone Has Something They Excel At

We're all excellent at something, and that's why comparisons to others, who have different talents and skill sets, are really not helpful. If you're still having trouble looking in the mirror, try this: Assess your physical strengths and weaknesses and focus on your strongest and best area. For some it's their shoulders; for others it's their legs. You will learn how to emphasize that region—whether it's how you dress, how you work out, or how you carry yourself. Start with what makes you feel good and we will build the foundation from there.

I take this approach with all my partners. I start my rehearsals with the basics—a cha-cha rocking forward step. This is just to see if my partner has some natural rhythm. If not, I immediately start to figure out what would look good on him. Maybe he's got strong, toned arms and broad shoulders, so I'll devise moves that will highlight his upper body and posture. Discovering what our partners excel at and then showcasing it is the job of all the professional dancers on *Dancing with the Stars*. We have to try to disguise the flaws and concentrate on the positives.

If, for example, you have strong arms and shoulders from carrying your baby or toddler around—and believe me, lifting your little ones is a great workout that you don't even think about!—then do those exercises first. They'll be easier for you, and you will see results more quickly. That will give you the confidence you need to work on the rest of your body.

And be sure to wear workout gear that highlights your best qualities. If your legs are strong and muscled, show them off in shorts. If your shoulders are shapely, wear sleeveless tops for exercise and off-the-shoulder tops when you go out. What matters most is that you have the confidence to feel good and highlight your assets with pride and grace.

Short Workouts Are Surprisingly Effective

All movement is good movement. You don't have to go to the gym for an hour or run for six miles every day to be an effective exerciser. It is much better to do at least one short workout every day than to do none. When your workouts make you feel good, you will be motivated to keep doing them. Because . . .

When You Start Small, It's So Much Easier to Reach Your Goals

Start slow. At least you're starting. If you only have two minutes today, do two perfect minutes. Maybe tomorrow you'll have three minutes. Next week you'll have ten. No matter how short or long your workout, realize that you always have another chance to do another one! Acknowledge the work you did, and be proud of yourself. Everyone starts somewhere!

Confidence Comes with Constant Repetition

Remember what I said in chapter 1 about toning your confidence? Confidence comes with repetition. My dance partners need to know that I am there for them and that with my teaching they may not get everything down the first day, but they will end up getting better. You break it down and the next day, guess what? You're actually doing it. It might not be technically great yet, but by the end of the week you're doing it and having fun and enjoying dancing.

That's why I think *Dancing with the Stars* is so popular—you see the progression each week with the celebrities, in real time. The audience watches familiar faces achieving things by doing them step by step, over and over again. Confidence begets confidence, and these non-dancers bloom as the weeks go by. There is absolutely no reason why you can't do the same!

Think of this when you're tackling the exercises in this book. When

Tips for Pre- or Postnatal Moms
from Dancer/Trainer Rockell Williamson-Rudder,
International Director of Xtend Barre

When you're pregnant, be smart with your choices and how you work out. Do what feels great, but don't for a moment worry about your tummy/abs staying flat and toned. Think more about stabilizing your body than doing a million crunches.

The same goes for postnatal. Let your body heal through restorative exercises, first under some private supervision by a professional, if possible, before jumping back into group classes at a gym or workouts on your own. I am always shocked at how little support is given to women who have had any pelvic dysfunction—it's very common. Speak to your doctor and start slow.

you do your first High Plank, if you can hold it for ten seconds, that's a lot! Every day you do another plank, and your muscles will strengthen. Before you know, you'll be holding a High Plank for an entire minute—something you never thought you'd be able to do. Your confidence will grow with repetition, so stick with the program!

My Workout Style

My workout style is very simple: I like to be comfy when I work out, but I still try to look cute! I like form-fitting workout tights, a good supportive workout bra, and a loose tank top. I'm a girl with curves and like to feel supported when working out so I don't bounce too much.

I recommend avoiding wearing any pants, shorts, or tights that don't fit properly. You want a wide range of motion and shouldn't ever be worried about people seeing your undies. Same for your bra. You don't want to be busting out or flopping about, and you can actually damage your breast tissue and cause sagging, without good support. Women with large breasts should look for compression-style workout bras as they help keep you in place comfortably.

Your workout shoes should also fit properly. Buy them in person, ideally from a sporting-goods store where the salespeople are knowledgeable. There are so many choices and it's so hard to know what is best for you, so never be afraid to ask an expert. I've tried to fit into shoes that were too small and it's not a good idea!

When wearing high heels I do like to put a cushion pad in the ball of my foot. For workouts, it's much more important to have a supportive shoe that fits perfectly, for the exercises or sport that you're doing, than to choose a pair because you like the color. And be sure to wear comfy socks that wick away moisture. Last but not least, I highly recommend investing in a pair of cozy slippers or Uggs for at home—you'll need them after all those workouts you'll be completing.

My Makeup Routine and Makeup Bag

When I go to the gym I don't like to wear too much makeup—just a little bit of light coverage. I wear a tinted moisturizer, which is a great item as it hydrates my skin while evening out my skin tone. A heavier foundation can clog your pores when you sweat—something all dancers know!—so I think it's best to let your skin breathe. Some tinted moisturizers also contain SPF, so you'll get light protection from the sun, too.

Also, I always curl my eyelashes and use a tinted lip balm or an Australian product called Lucas' Papaw Ointment. It's made from fermented Australian pawpaw and we love it—it's actually great as a skin soother and can be used on scrapes or rashes. It's perfect to have in your handbag.

I find that I am on the go a lot, so I do always have eyeliner; a neutral, light-colored lipstick; and pressed powder in my handbag in case I have to race off somewhere after my workouts.

My makeup bag itself has all the essentials: primer, foundation, tinted moisturizer (sometimes, for less heavy coverage, I mix tinted moisturizer and foundation on the back of my hand and then apply that with my fingertips or a makeup sponge), bronzer, an eyelash curler, mascara, an eyebrow pencil (that really gives your face a polished look), and a cream blush that can be used for lips and eye shadow as well.

My Skin-Care Routine

The makeup I have to wear for television and stage performances is much heavier and more opaque than my regular makeup. We dancers know how important it is to cleanse our faces really well—particularly after we've sweated all day. My mum also always told me to take my makeup off before I go to bed. As tired as I may be, it's something I always do. Always. Heavy makeup + sweat + the dirt of being in studio air = clogged pores and adult acne.

In the morning, for my face, I always moisturize and wear a non-oily SPF 30+ sunscreen under my foundation. We are very sun-conscious in Australia because it's so easy to get burned, and that got me into the good habit of keeping sunscreen on hand at all times. I also believe in a good night cream and an eye cream. I find a hydrating mask helps, too, at least once a month. I should get facials more often for deep cleansing, but I find I don't have the time. At-home facials can be nearly as effective, and they're a wonderful way to help you relax while waiting for the masks to dry as you watch TV or maybe even treat yourself to a glass of wine!

For my body, I use a lot of fake tanning products when on *Dancing with the Stars*, so I need to do a really good scrub before I apply it or it can get streaky. I use my favorite foot scrub (see the next section) all over my body. At night I like to mix coconut oil with moisturizer to apply before I go to bed. It makes my skin soft and smells really good, too!

Know Your Limits So You Don't Get Injured

Professional dancers develop a high tolerance for pain. Our bodies are the foundation of our work, so it's inevitable that there will be minor injuries, like cuts, scrapes, and sprains, or major ones, with torn muscles or broken bones that can have a catastrophic effect on our careers. I've been fortunate to have had few injuries—in part because I always like to warm up—but the handful of bad ones were real doozies!

When I was doing *Burn the Floor* I tore the ligaments in my ankle. We were in Austria at the time and I had to leave the tour and fly back to Australia and have some intensive physical therapy. I was devastated and felt that I had let everyone down, but we all knew that these things happen. I was lucky I didn't need surgery, and I got myself better with physical therapy.

Then, when I was doing the *Dancing with the Stars* tour, I fractured my knuckle when I was walking down the stairs and trying to be super sexy. On the fifth step I lost my balance and fell. I literally did a dive off the stage. I knew that if I fell straight down I'd hit my head, so I managed to land on my knuckle (of all things!) instead and it broke.

Luckily, Drew Lachey was on the tour, and he was standing right there. He used to be a paramedic, so he looked after me until I got to the hospital. There wasn't much they could do for me, and I've had problems with it ever since as there's a lot of bad scar tissue. Even now, I have to be diligent about stretching out my fingers and doing some hand strengthening exercises for grip strength or my hand gets really stiff. Like my mum says, "You just have to keep moving. When you stop moving, that's when things stop working!"

The worst injury of my career to date happened in 2011 while I was competing on *Dancing with the Stars* with Hines Ward, who's an elite athlete and a great football player. We'd made it to the semifinals, and at that stage everything becomes even more competitive and you want to do things that haven't been done on the show before for that wow factor. I thought if there was ever a chance for me to do something different with some incredible lifts, it would be with this amazingly strong football player. So I was trying a quite dangerous lift that I'd seen some world salsa champions do—which was pretty stupid on my part because I forgot that Hines wasn't a trained dancer with years of experience doing complicated lifts. I could teach him as much as I knew, and we got it right a few times. But for the fateful lift, we didn't have the correct momentum, and he lost his balance and fell on top of me, with his whole body weight crushing my neck. I instantly went numb to my elbows and was trying very hard not to panic, because I knew it was a really bad injury. I felt like I wanted to throw up and I knew that wasn't good, either. Some of the other dancers came rushing in, and Hines was great in looking after me; he'd seen many of his fellow football players get injured on the field. The ambulance turned up really quickly and braced my neck and put me on the stretcher. Once we got to the ER, the neurosurgeons weren't quite sure what had happened, and the producers had been smart enough to come to the hospital (with Hines, who was devastated with worry), and show them the footage. They were shocked that I wasn't paralyzed, and they told me I needed an immediate MRI to check my head and neck. They asked if I had any metal on, and I told them my dance shoes. They lifted up the sheets and there were my three-and-a-half-inch heels sticking out!

I was very, very lucky. My neck bones were bruised and my spinal cord was sprained, and I'd also torn some ligaments in my neck. The doctors told me that the tear was what saved me, because the torn ligaments swelled up so quickly that they cushioned the bones so they didn't fracture. When Hines fell on top of me it was like it happened in slow motion, just like other accident victims say it does. It was so slow when he fell on me that I went limp and I went with it instead of stiffening up. So I think that's what saved me, too.

I wasn't able to rehearse for a few days, so Cheryl Burke, one of my best friends on the show, stepped in and helped. But the competitor in me came out and I was determined to dance with Hines. We'd worked so hard and gotten so far, and I got through it! My doctors weren't happy with me, and they told me that if I had been a basketball or football player, they would have forbidden me to get to work. Fortunately, I don't think they fully understood what dancers actually do, and how intense the work and the movement is. I was on quite a lot of heavy painkillers, and we changed a few of the steps in the routine because I couldn't move my neck back and forward or fully extend. I was rehearsing with the brace, and doing a lot of physical therapy, but I took it off to do the show. It was even more satisfying than usual to make it to the finals. Coming back from that injury to win the Mirror Ball trophy that year with Hines was one of my most memorable dance moments ever. I'd practically had to break my neck to win that trophy!

Still, it took me a long time to fully heal, and my neck still gives me a little bit of a problem. I have arthritis there now, which is actually very common for dancers but might have been triggered by the injury. When I stopped taking painkillers after the show, I felt like I'd been hit by a truck. It was pretty intense. I had to take a few months off and do a lot of physical therapy to ease myself back into dancing, but I luckily didn't need surgery for this injury either.

What did I learn after this injury? I pushed myself and my partner too far. I did something risky that I shouldn't have attempted. I knew better, but in the heat of the moment, I let my competitive drive get the better of my common sense. It was a very painful lesson for me, physically and emotionally. I could have ended my career then and been gravely injured.

Always be aware of your limits. You should feel the exercises in your muscles when you work out, and you should feel the stretches when you do them, but never to the point of pain. If something hurts, stop. "No pain, no gain" is a total fallacy! Assess your form and be sure you're doing the move correctly. If it still hurts for any reason, stop. Only move on to more reps or more difficult exercises when you've mastered the basics. As you know already, when you start small, you work out effectively, with little risk of pain or injury.

And no risky lifts, please!

Have a Positive Mind-set and Be Kind to Yourself

Please do not beat yourself up if you miss a few days of exercising or just don't feel like it. You know what you need to do, and you'll do it! I've had plenty of days where I felt awful, especially as it's always difficult to be judged and get bad scores. Not only does that leave me frustrated with myself, but I feel extra-terrible for my partners. It's up to me to put on a smile, turn whatever happened into a positive, and get going for another week.

So I never want you to say things like, "Oh, I'm so bad. I can't believe I haven't worked out in such a long time and I just ate a whole bag of potato chips."

Instead, flip the narrative and be positive. Say, "Well, I enjoyed that time off. Tomorrow is a new day and a fresh start, and I'm going to make the most of it." Then move on.

My partners learned how to move on right away—as soon as they finished the performance of the week. "Time to throw that one out the window!" I'd tell them. "It doesn't matter if you missed a few steps or it was the best dance you ever did. It's gone. Forget about it. It's time to concentrate on the next dance."

Sometimes I'd get a few grumbles, especially when they received great scores for the routine and wanted to celebrate, but a day or two later we'd be working so hard on the next dance, the previous one really was forgotten.

Florence Henderson on Fitness and Dancing

No matter your age it's important to respect your body and know how your body works. I've been in the business forever and I was known as the singer who could move. I could learn dances quickly but never had any formal training, so I had no idea how difficult and meticulous ballroom dancing was. In fact, I've worked out all my life—at least three times a week, on my own or sometimes with a trainer. In addition, I walk on the treadmill, ride the exercise bike, or I do Pilates and a mix of weights. If I hadn't done that I would never have lasted six weeks on *Dancing with the Stars*.

I was most nervous about learning the dances. Once I got in there and understood the nuances of ballroom dancing, I realized how easy the pros made it seem—but It was so hard. I was also worried about stamina. Kym would always be willing to come in to help Corky and me when we were training. I struggled with the quick step and tango, but when I saw Kym get so badly injured in her season with Hines Ward and still be able to get up and regroup and push forward, it was an inspiration to me that I could continue even when I was starting to feel bumped up and bruised. I did a lot of big Broadway shows when I first started my career and *Dancing with the Stars* was just like that— you rehearse so hard and you hope you embody the right character to bring the story to life for the audience. It's live, and you have to be ready to perform. You get butterflies in your stomach when the music starts, and since it's live there's no turning back—if you fall, you fall!

I took part in the *Dancing with the Stars: At Sea* cruises in 2015, so I had to get in good shape. I maintained my three workouts per week, with a focus on cardio. I also did more walking outside, doing different speed intervals to make sure my stamina was high.

This is a wonderful strategy for everything in life. Holding on to the past keeps you stuck in it. Learn from your triumphs as well as your disappointments, but don't let them rule your present or your future. Otherwise, it's much harder to move on.

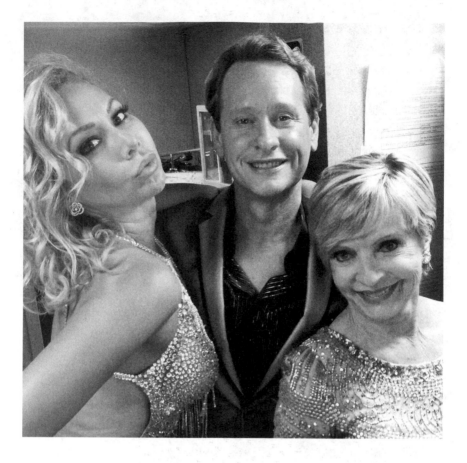

Be Creative: Choreograph Your Own Unique Workout

You're going to get very comfortable doing all of the movements and exercises you'll see in the next few chapters. Once you master them—which will take so much less time than you think!—you can pick and choose your routines and customize the workouts you like. Some people thrive on routine and always do the same sequence, as it makes them feel comfortable. If that's you, great! If you need a lot of change to keep things fresh, that's great, too!

A super-easy way to change up your workout is simply to switch your starting side. Most people are right-handed and naturally start on the right. If you force yourself to start on your left, you will be surprised at first how much more difficult it is. Everyone has a dominant side,

Great Advice from Rockell Williamson-Rudder

When I was in my twenties, as a professional dancer, working out never felt like it had that title as such because conditioning would be centered around doing classes, rehearsals, or showtime. It felt rather easy to stay fit, and I never felt like I was working out as I simply loved to move my body through dance and lived and breathed it all day, every day.

That doesn't mean that the expectations placed on my body as a pro dancer weren't at times extreme both physically and emotionally, so I wish I knew then what I know now that I'm in my late thirties. I would have been a healthier, stronger dancer—I am certain of that. To any young dancers out there, read and learn what you can about how your body actually moves/works and embrace what knowledge you can about nourishing your body with the right fuel. The fuel someone else uses for their body may not be what your body needs. There is no such thing as a diet. Experiment with what works for you.

Three children later and no longer performing, I certainly need something that keeps my body strong inside and out. I am blessed that after a career in entertainment I now work in the fitness industry, and I'm fortunate to know how best to nurture my joints as they get older, prepare for pre- and postnatal care and restoration; and, as a busy working mum, equip myself to be fit and healthy for my family. Interestingly, I have never felt stronger and more in control of my body.

For me, working out needs to not feel like working out—it has to be in a class environment that is fun and electric, with an instructor who makes me want to work hard for them. Before I know it, I have done an hour of training and had a good time! I also call working out my moving meditation as my mind really does switch off from what-

and that side is always stronger and more coordinated. Using more of your nondominant side will not only strengthen the muscles there but improve your coordination.

I can tell you how true this is from experience. When I'm with my partners on *Dancing with the Stars*, I'm teaching the men and doing their steps. Those steps are the opposite of mine. I have to know the male and ever else is going on in my life and I just relish the good endorphins. If for whatever reason I miss chances to work out, I can feel my mind and body get sluggish.

Staying motivated is tough though, I totally get it, so try to find a studio or gym that offers more than a class. It should be a place where you can meet some friends old or new, and work out with people who empower you. It also helps you be accountable, so arrange to meet someone to train with.

Tips for keeping on track with your workout schedule: Book yourself into your calendar for an hour each day. Make that hour a time when you attend a class or something just for you. Prepay for your classes or pass so that you don't cancel or it costs you money! Be kind to yourself.

Tips for traveling: Download an app that has your favorite workouts on it so you can follow them at the hotel or wherever you are. Stretch! The best thing after a long flight is to spend thirty minutes stretching every part of your body. Use a towel if you need to, as it will help the stretching. You will have less jet lag if you don't eat too much and then sit still on a long-haul flight. Don't be afraid to do some moves and stretches a couple of times during the flight. Yes, I am that girl who does pliés in the aisles! I always find the local supermarket as soon as I land somewhere to stock up on a few things, even if it is just some nuts, carrots, and hummus to have at the hotel.

At the end of the day and across over three decades, it has always come down to one thing in my life . . . and that is the positive influence dance can have on your body. Whether that is in a dance fitness class, a ballroom social class, or ballet classes, moving your body to some great music is fun and feels good.

female parts, all the time, and be able to effortlessly switch back and forth. It keeps me on my toes—literally! And when I was shooting my exercise DVDs, I had to do all the moves starting on the left side for the camera, so everyone at home would see the reverse and start on their right. I really had to think about what I was doing!

Make It Fun

My *Dancing with the Stars* partner Joey Fatone has this to say about enjoying yourself on the dance floor: "Kym was always calm and cool when teaching me, and I'm always trying to outdo myself and be the best I can be. I think I helped her—kidding!—on the first show of season four. Right before we went out, I said, 'Hey, let's just have fun. Screw everything else!'"

Joey knew, as I do, that one of the reasons dancing is such a joy is because we move to music. If I'm running on a treadmill I find that it can be very difficult if I don't have any music, but as soon as I put on the headphones, I don't even think I'm working out. I become the music and I'm dancing. Even if I'm walking, running, or cycling, music makes me feel like I'm dancing. That's why dancing is such a great workout. You don't feel like you're working out at all. You're just enjoying what you're doing and moving to the music.

I can't think of a better way to bring fun into your life than putting on some songs that will get your toes tapping and your spirit filled with happiness. My mum is seventy-four years old and she loves to dance socially. She's a great role model. She looks incredible, and she has the body of a thirty-year-old (seriously!). She makes sure that she's moving, every single day. And she also loves it, which makes a big difference. Her friends love it, too. I've seen them when they go out dancing, and they're always laughing and singing along to the songs, and the time just flies by. In the meantime they've burned hundreds of calories and toned their entire bodies without even thinking about it.

Whatever kind of exercise you're drawn to, you're much more likely to stick to it if you really love it.

Carson Kressley on Having Fun

I had no professional dance training before I went on the show—and it showed! Still, I was in pretty good shape before I started and surprisingly athletic and flexible from years and years of equestrian competitions. I rehearsed about six hours a day, which is the best exercise, because you are working out without really thinking that you are working out. My favorite!

Then I usually did core strengthening and flexibility exercises with a fabulous retired Russian prima ballerina who had been with the Ballets Russes—in total about eight hours of exercise every day for six weeks. Needless to say I was in the best shape of my life and could eat anything!

After the first rehearsal, I was absolutely overwhelmed. There is so much to learn and so little time to learn it. Eventually you just get down to doing the work and focusing on your routine. I didn't really worry about the competition. I just worried about me doing my best. And it worked! Although the actual dancing was hard. I'm just not a natural.

Doing the very first routine was the most nerve-wracking thing ever—like taking your driver's test times a million! My biggest fear was forgetting my entire routine. It happens. And praise the Lord it didn't happen to me! I just kept telling myself, *There's no time for that. You gotta just keep moving!* No one ever knew that I would go so into my "zone" that I never even really heard the music. I would just dance step to step chronologically until the routine was over. I'm a bit of a savant that way.

Still, I just really tried to enjoy the process and remember how lucky I was to be working with a world-class dancer. I made it more about enjoying the process than the final result. The routines almost never go off perfectly. I tried to focus on what we did right. Pure enthusiasm for the dance and also wanting to entertain the crowd helped a lot. I channeled my inner Shirley Temple.

I try to keep dancing—it's the greatest exercise because you are distracted by the steps, the music, and the fun of it. I hate to work out, so something that tricks me like dance does is great for me. Although I didn't dance with Kym on the show, we have worked together on other dance shows like *Dancing with the Stars: At Sea*—a fan cruise for lovers of the show. I think the most memorable thing about Kym's coaching is the positivity she radiates. With her you just believe you can do anything and she breaks it down to digestible steps that are achievable.

Buddy Up! Find a Workout Partner

Another great way to make exercise fun is to buddy up. Sometimes I'm in a contemplative mood and just want to be on my own when I work out.

Other times I'm feeling social and want to have a friend with me. Having company always makes the time fly by. You can talk and laugh and encourage each other, or you can train hard and not say much, just give subtle encouragement and push yourselves for a superlative session. On our tour, Whitney, Emma, and I would jump rope, do some core exercises, and run around the stadium before we performed. Then when we'd get to the hotel we'd go for a workout. It was so nice to have partners in crime to help me push myself and keep me motivated when I was on the road.

Just make sure your workout buddy is as committed as you are. If you grow dependent on each other, when one person has to cancel, it's easy to use that as an excuse not to do a solo workout!

Don't Get Bored, Get Busy!

The best teachers are always learning from their students. I learned from every one of my partners on *Dancing with the Stars*; each was unique. Some people asked me if I ever got bored after so many seasons, but that was never the case. On the contrary—every celebrity had a different personality, and their needs and talents brought out something new in me every time. The challenge for me was to figure out what would bring out their best, too. I had to adapt my teaching style to them. And I learned that the best teachers don't just do what they know and what's easy for them. They assess the situation and they adapt. And when that happens, you are never bored!

There's another kind of boredom, too, and that's what happens when you might not like what you're doing (endless paperwork at the office, for example) and you feel like you're in a rut. When I'm feeling that way I tend to reach for the closest snack in sight. I want to distract myself with anything at all—including food. Now, if I find myself feeling bored or restless with chores, I do a few core or other exercises instead. If you try that, not only will you have ignored what's in the kitchen or in the snack room at the office, but you will have toned your muscles, improved your circulation, burned some calories, improved your energy, and made an excellent choice that will fill you with well-earned pride and satisfaction. You will soon learn to associate movement with feeling good, and boredom will be nothing more than a passing memory.

Reward Yourself

Another way to stave off boredom or predictability is to reward yourself. In fact, you can start giving yourself treats as soon as you master one of the exercises in this book. The first time you hold a High Plank for more than ten or twenty seconds is worthy of celebration. Your treat can be as simple as a phone call to someone for encouragement. It could be a facial or a massage or a new lipstick or a book. It could be a gold star on your refrigerator so your kids can see how hard you are working. And when you drop a dress size, you certainly should go celebrate by buying yourself a wonderful new outfit.

The point is, you need to acknowledge your determination and goals. You deserve the best—and if you don't give it to yourself, who will?

Let Your Light Shine

I always told my partners on the show that the first time we went out to the floor in front of the live audience, we needed to do something to stand out. Even if you're not the best technical dancer, the audience wants to watch you perform and have fun. I've danced with celebrities who may not have mastered the footwork, but the fans really supported them because they brought their personality and passion for the dance to life.

When I was rehearsing with Robert Herjavec—an incredibly successful businessman and entrepreneur, and a leading investor on ABC's reality series *Shark Tank*—I told him that he had to sell every dance. He looked at me and smiled. "It's so funny you say that, because when I do *Shark Tank* I'm sitting there saying to all of these people that they need to do something to stand out to separate themselves from the rest," he said. "And I feel like that's what you need to do as a dancer. To let your light shine in a big way."

So that's what I said to him before every performance. "Let your light shine, you can do this."

You need to find the mantra that will work to motivate you. Write it down, post it on the wall in front of where you work out—whatever it takes to refer back to those words of inspiration, so you keep pushing yourself to continue.

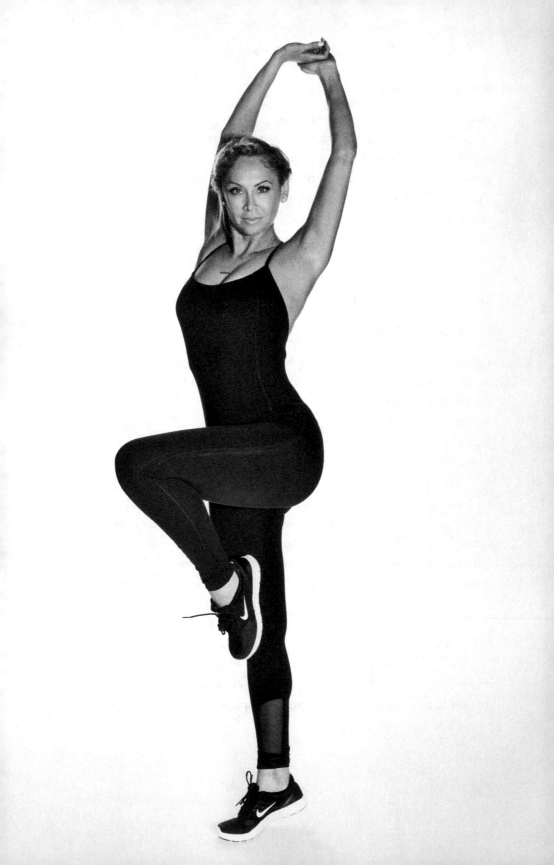

7

The Core Workouts

As a dancer, I learned at a very early age that posture is key. From little girls in tutus doing port de bras (which means, literally, "carriage of the arms") to ballroom dancers taking the first steps of the rumba walk, having a strong core is the foundation for all movement in dance. All the training that a dancer goes through will always relate back to having a strong core.

Most people think that their core is only the abdominal muscles that support the belly area. That's not quite right—your core is actually the entire center of your body. It consists of your abdominal muscles, as well as those in the lower back, hips, and pelvic floor. It's better to think of it as three-dimensional, because the core muscles in your front are as important as the core muscles of your back. Time to bust a popular myth—you can't do crunches every day and expect to develop a strong core. I have some friends who love to go to the gym and run but neglect to focus on their core. They are super fit and have great stamina but quite often suffer from lower back pain and bad posture. I also have a friend who just loves to lift weights—and he does look extremely nice and toned in his board shorts—but his muscles are so overdeveloped that they tend to stress his back and hip muscles from time to time. Good core training helps you develop all of your stabilizers, and that's where the good posture comes from!

Being a dancer has given me an understanding of how important core strength is, not only for dancing but also in everyday life, especially as I get older. I feel a difference in my body when I don't focus on my core. On *Dancing with the Stars*, it was the first thing I looked at when a new celebrity walked in the door to start a new season with me. Don't get me wrong, I didn't ask them to lift up their shirt and show me their abs right off the bat! We'd turn on the music and start with some basic movements, and I'd be watching their balance to gauge how strong their core was. That's when I'd really start to recognize what I was dealing with! I tell anyone I train with that without a good core, you won't be able to control the movement of the dance.

Now, not everyone believes this at first, but some of my famous sporting partners are the biggest advocates for my "core first" approach. These athletes are usually amazed at the fitness level of all the professional dancers on the show. They compare us to any elite athlete—quite rightly, too! Some have even taken what they learned on the dance floor and applied it to their own sport. My wonderful partner Hines Ward was going straight back to his team, the Pittsburgh Steelers, after we won the Mirror Ball in 2011. He said dancing was the best preseason training he's ever done. Plus, he ended up with some pretty smooth touchdown moves, too!

I like to begin any dance rehearsal with a quick core workout just like the ones I've designed for this chapter. It's the perfect way to start connecting with my partner and make sure we are activating the core so we are ready to start moving. My core workouts have become well-known by the entire cast on *Dancing with the Stars*. At the training facility, a lot of competitors have joined in my morning core sessions; especially when we're on tour, we like to warm up for any show together by doing a five-minute abs session. Most of the time this ends with us in laughing fits backstage when we should have been concentrating on our breathing—but the point is, even then we are engaging the core!

These are the basic benefits of core training:

- improves whole-body strength and performance

- helps prevent injuries

- can improve respiratory function

- improves posture

- often improves or alleviates lower back pain, which is often caused by bad posture

- tightens and flattens your stomach and lower abdomen

- improves your balance, which can help prevent falls and injuries

- improves your agility

- improves overall strength

With a strong core, everyday activities you likely don't even think about become so much easier: bending to tie your shoes, taking a shower, dressing, sitting in a chair, turning your head to look behind you when you're driving, or even just standing still will become simpler for you to do.

By now, you shouldn't need any more convincing . . . It all starts with the core!

You just need a few minutes each day to get your core in great shape. And there's no downside to doing these exercises every day.

So let's get started!

How to Breathe When Doing Your Core Workouts

Your breathing muscles are also part of your core muscles. This makes it vital that you use proper breathing techniques while performing core-strengthening exercises so that you can optimize the results of the movement. Never hold your breath! It's important to take full breaths in through the nose and out through the mouth. As the exercises become more challenging, your breath rate will change. Remember to breathe at your own pace, but focus on taking full breaths, in and out.

1. THREE-MINUTE WORKOUT: CORE QUICKIE

These are easy-to-learn exercises that automatically engage your core muscles. Do them whenever you have three minutes and you will be surprised at how quickly they'll tone you up!

Total Time: Three minutes.

Equipment Needed: An exercise mat, towel, or soft surface.

What to Do: Perform these three abdominal exercises for one minute each.

Basic Crunch

1. Lie flat on your back with your feet flat on the ground and your knees bent.

2. Place your hands lightly on either side of your head, with your elbows pointing away from your ears.

3. Slowly begin to roll your shoulders off the floor and tighten your abs as you lift. Your shoulders should only come up off the floor about four inches. Be sure to keep your feet flat on the floor.

4. Control the release on the way down.

TIPS
- Use your muscles, not momentum. You should feel it in your abs.

- Do not arch your back or pull on your neck when going up.

- Exhale on the way up and inhale on the way down.

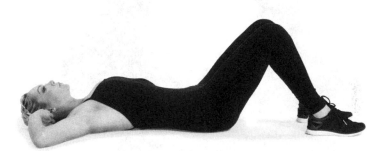

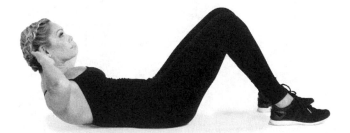

Windshield-Wiper Legs

1. Lie flat on your back with your legs up, extended over your hips, and your hands pressing into the floor.

2. Slowly lower your legs toward one side, back to center, then to the other side.

TIP
If you feel any strain in your back, bend your knees while you continue the movement.

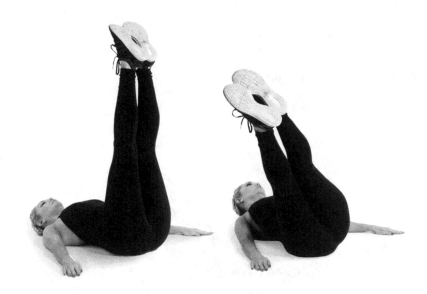

Bicycle Crunch

1. Lie flat on your back with your lower back pressed to the ground.

2. Place your hands beside your head, with elbows pointing away from your ears, and lift your shoulders into a crunch position.

3. Bring your knees up toward your chest. Knees should be perpendicular to the floor, with your lower legs parallel to the floor.

4. Slowly go through a bicycle-pedal motion, kicking forward with the right leg and keeping the knee of the left leg in toward your chest. Bring your right elbow close to your left knee by crunching to the side, then switch to the opposite side by extending the left leg and taking the left elbow to the right knee.

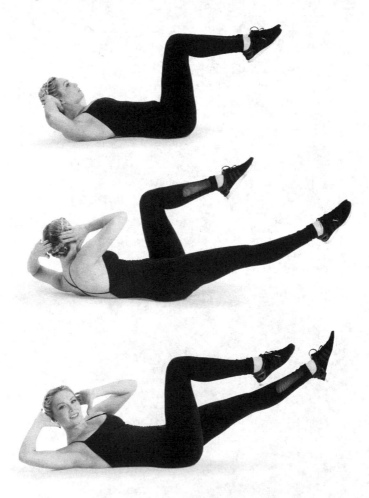

2. Five-Minute Workout: Total Core

This five-minute workout is more challenging because I'm adding some balance elements. Here you'll be working the glutes as well as your lower back in addition to the abdominals. Remember to think of the entire center of your body as your core—you have to focus on more than just your abs. It may be tough to balance at first, but stick with it—the more you repeat the movement, the stronger your stabilizers will become!

Total Time: Five minutes.

Equipment Needed: An exercise mat, towel, or soft surface.

What to Do: Perform these five exercises for one minute each.

Bird Dog

1. Position yourself on all fours with your shoulders over your wrists and your hips over your knees.

2. Raise one arm to shoulder height while simultaneously extending the opposite leg to hip height.

3. Slowly lower your arm and leg at the same time.

4. Alternate sides.

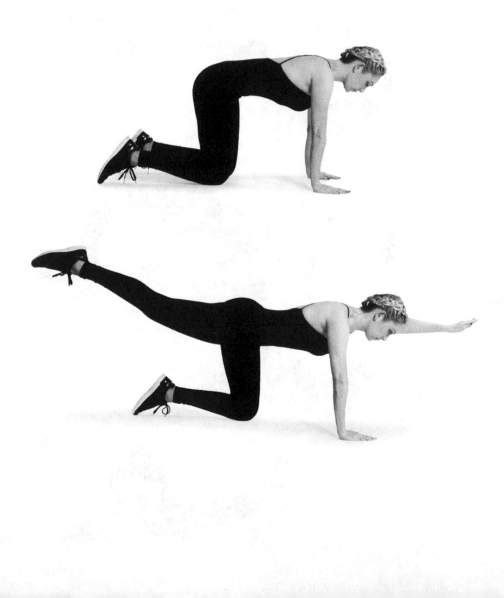

Hip Bridge to Crunch

1. Lie flat on your back with your hands by your sides and your knees bent. Your feet should be shoulder-width apart.

2. Pushing mainly with your heels, lift your hips off the floor while keeping your back straight.

3. Squeeze your glutes at the top.

4. Lower your hips back to the floor.

5. Place your hands behind your head and perform a Basic Crunch (page 161).

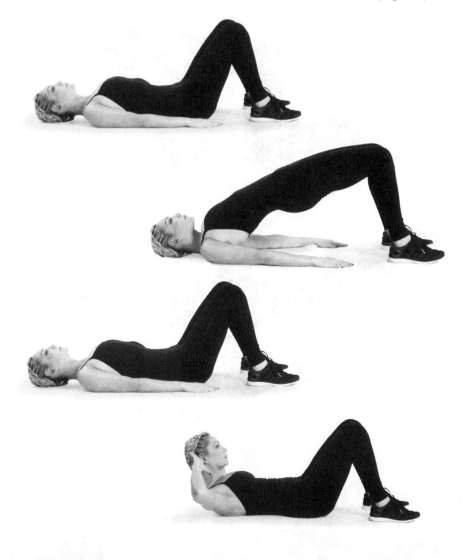

Straight-Leg Drops

1. Lie flat on your back with your lower back pressed to the ground.

2. Place your hands beside your head, with your elbows pointing away from your ears, and lift your shoulders into the Basic Crunch (page 161) position.

3. Keeping your legs straight, raise your right leg straight up and your left leg straight out in front of you. Your legs should be creating an L shape.

4. Slowly switch the position of the legs from one side to the other.

TIP
If you feel any strain in your back, slightly bend your knees.

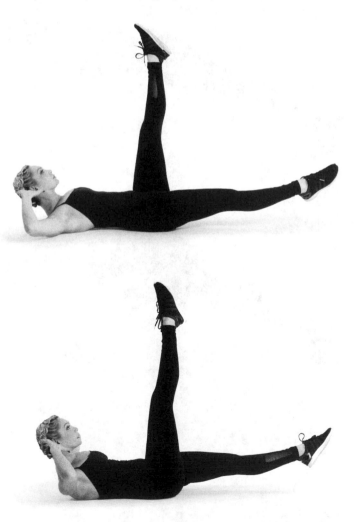

Plank Knee Pulls

1. Start in a High Plank position. See page 170 for instructions.

2. Lift your right leg off the floor and pull your knee toward your left elbow.

3. Return your right leg back to starting position and repeat on the left side.

TIP
You can start out just holding the High Plank and gradually build up to moving your knees.

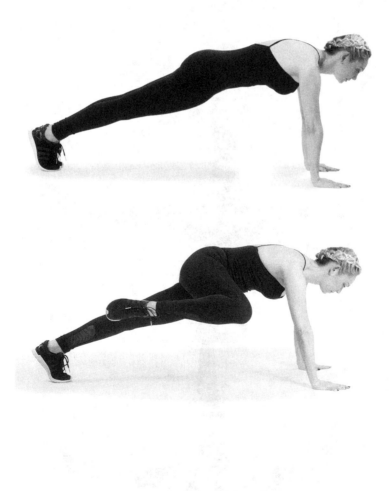

Back Extensions

1. Lie facedown with your arms extended, fingertips or palms flat on the floor.

2. Squeezing your glutes and lower back, raise your chest and legs two to six inches off the floor. Look up while you complete this movement.

3. Slowly release and return your chest and legs to the floor.

TIP
Be sure to keep your legs straight the entire time.

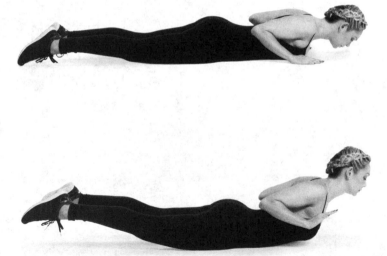

3. Five-Minute Workout: Rock the Plank

Of all the exercises you can do, a plank is by far one of the best. It might look deceptively easy when you see someone in this position, but because it engages so many of your muscles at once—giving you a full-body workout—it's one of the best exercises you can do.

Don't expect to be able to do this entire routine smoothly the first time you try it, especially if you've never done planks before. Do as much as you can. Then, each time you repeat the sequence, you'll get better at it.

Total Time: Five minutes.

Equipment Needed: An exercise mat, towel, or soft surface.

What to Do: Your goal is to hold each plank for thirty seconds, take a fifteen-second rest, and then move right into the next plank variation.

High Plank

1. Lie facedown on the floor, then push through your hands to lift up your entire body in a straight line. You should be comfortably supporting your weight on your toes and hands.

2. Hold this position.

TIPS
• Keep your shoulders over your wrists.

• Keep your glutes (the muscles in your butt) and abs tight while maintaining this position. It's essential to keep your body perfectly straight, because if you sag in the middle or raise your butt up too high, your core will not get the workout it needs!

• Newbies to the plank or those with any lower back issues can start out with a Half Plank. Let your knees stay on the floor; you'll look like you're about to do a push-up. Be sure to keep your back straight.

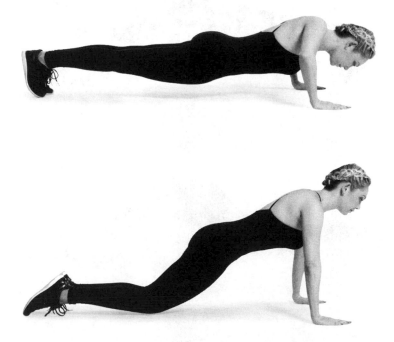

Elbow Plank

1. Lie facedown on the floor, then push your body up into a straight line with your weight on your toes and hands.

2. Come down onto your elbows, which should be directly under your shoulders, with your forearms extended in front of you and your palms facedown on the floor.

3. You should be comfortably supporting your weight on your toes and forearms.

4. Squeeze your abs and glutes, keeping your hips lifted. Hold this position.

TIPS

- Keep your shoulders over your elbows.

- As with the High Plank, you can modify this plank by lowering your knees to the floor.

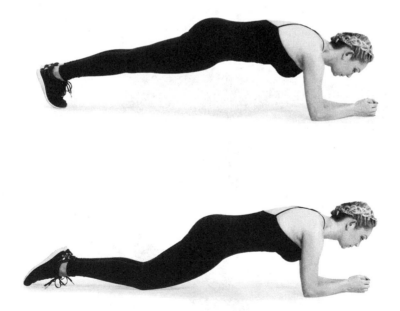

High Plank + Oblique Knee Pulls

1. Start in the High Plank position.

2. Lift your right leg off the floor and pull your knee toward your right elbow. Return leg back to starting position.

3. Repeat on the left side.

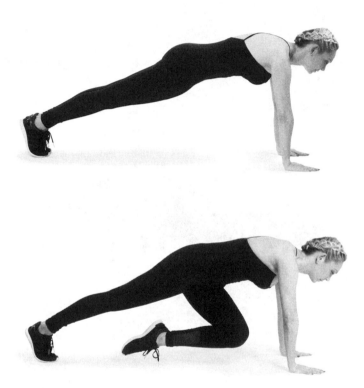

Side Plank

1. Lie on your side with your elbow directly beneath your shoulder.

2. Supporting yourself on your forearm, push your body up into a straight line, raising your hips and extending your opposite arm straight up.

3. Squeeze your feet and knees together.

4. Keeping your abs and glutes tight, hold this position.

5. Switch sides.

TIP
As with the High Plank, you can modify this plank by lowering your knees to the floor.

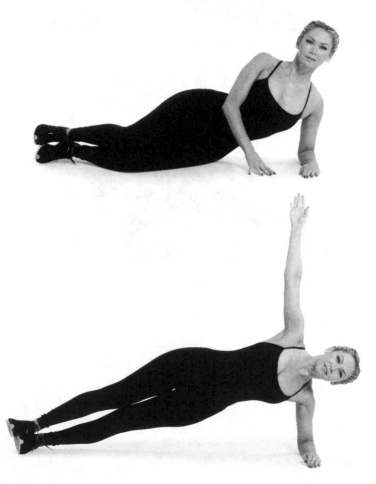

Plank Cinch

1. Start in the Elbow Plank (page 171) position.

2. Keep your feet and knees together, and rock your hips from side to side, dropping one hip toward the floor at a time.

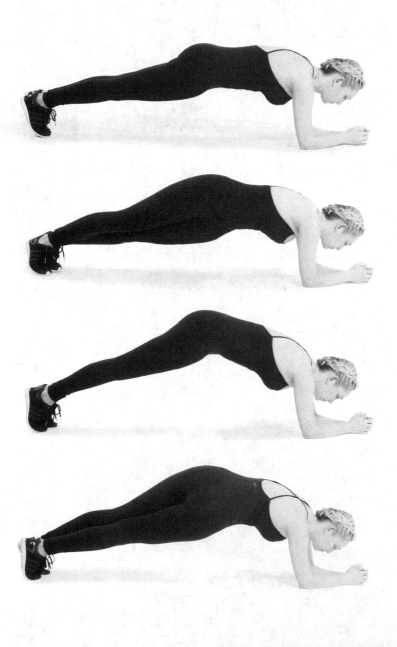

4. Six-Minute Workout: Standing Core

Taking your core routine off the ground and onto your feet gives you more bang for your buck. While you're standing, your core muscles instantly turn on; they act as stabilizers to keep you upright. That means that as soon as you begin the exercises on your feet, your core muscles are targeting twice as much because they are already activated! An even bigger bonus—you are burning more calories upright than you would lying down.

I love these exercises, because they can be done anywhere. If you find yourself dragging while you're hard at work behind a desk, then get up and spend six minutes doing them—you can even have your colleagues join in. You'll feel super energized afterward, and your abs will thank you!

Total Time: Six minutes.

Equipment Needed: None.

What to Do: Perform these five standing exercises for one minute each, except for the Jive Crunch, which takes two minutes (one minute per side).

Waistline Reach

1. Start standing with feet hip-width apart and arms by your sides.

2. Bending at the waist, reach to one side and then the other.

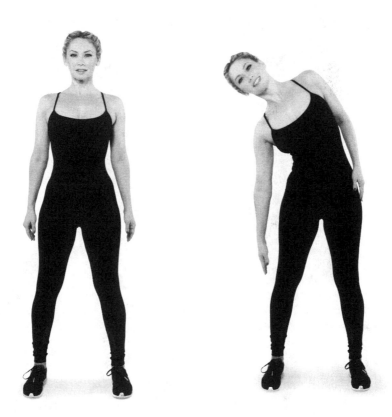

Jive Crunch

1. Start standing with feet hip-width apart.

2. Lift your right knee to your left elbow and crunch your abs.

3. Continue for one minute.

4. Repeat with your left knee and right elbow.

5. Continue for one minute.

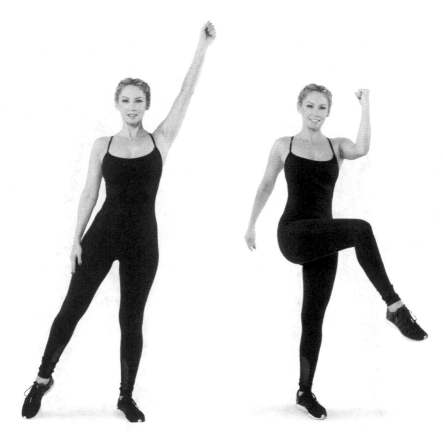

Dancer Isolations

1. Start standing with feet hip-width apart and arms stretched out at shoulder height.

2. Reach to one side with your right arm, then back to center.

3. Continue shifting side to side, controlling your movement back to center each time.

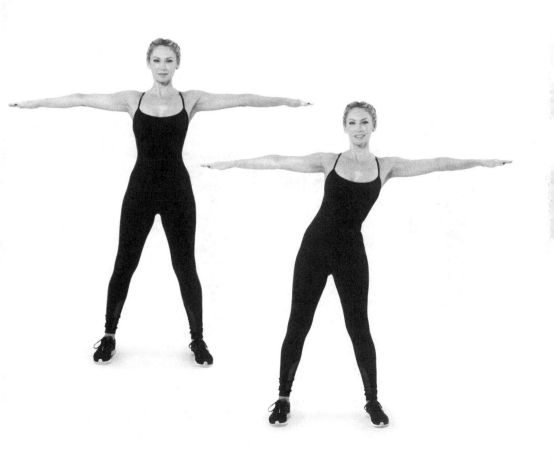

Pendulums

1. Start standing with feet hip-width apart.

2. With your arms extended straight overhead, hinge forward, lifting your back leg off the floor, creating a T position (also known as Warrior 3, for you yogis).

3. Maintain a straight line from the tip of your fingers to your toes and return to standing position.

4. Alternate sides.

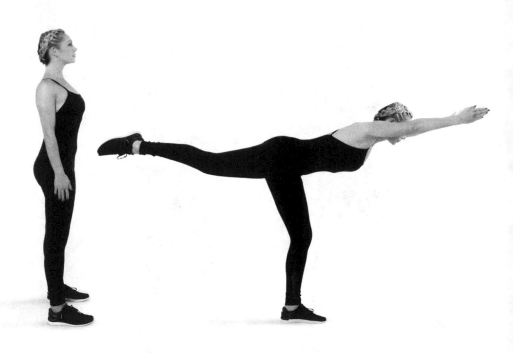

Latin Hip Rolls

1. Start standing with feet hip-width apart.

2. Make five hip circles to the right.

3. Make five hip circles to the left.

4. Continue alternating sides.

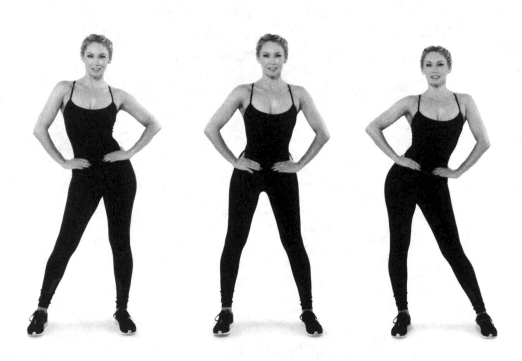

5. Sixteen-Minute Workout: Core Blast

This ultimate core workout combines my favorite standing exercises, crunches, back work, and glutes work from all the routines in this chapter that you've mastered so far. This is the ultimate core-strengthening and belly-fat-burning combination—so get ready to sweat.

Total Time: Sixteen minutes.

Equipment Needed: An exercise mat, towel, or soft surface.

What to Do: Perform these sixteen exercises for one minute each. Do them in the order listed, as they have been designed this way for maximum efficiency.

CORE BLAST

Basic Crunch

High Plank + Oblique Knee Pulls

Jive Crunch

Back Extensions

Latin Hip Rolls

Straight-Leg Drops

Pendulums

Elbow Plank

Bicycle Crunch

Plank Cinch

Waistline Reach

Bird Dog

Windshield-Wiper Legs

Dancer Isolations

Hip Bridge to Crunch

High Plank

8

Five-Minute Basics

When I'm traveling for performances I get the opportunity to meet so many fans of dance—people who love movement, music, and, of course, dance as much as I do! We also talk about health and fitness, and I find the discussion always comes around to our lack of time. Everyone is super busy—that can't be avoided—but you owe it to yourself to focus on moving. Any bit of movement you can do each day is great, and it's important to keep with it so it becomes part of your daily routine.

I kept those conversations in mind as I designed the exercises for this chapter. I want to make your workouts as fun and easy to incorporate into your day as possible. I've broken them down here into small five-minute blocks so you can see effective results while still fitting them into your schedule.

Here's what you need to know about my five-minute workouts:

- Each of these mini-routines targets a specific area. The elements take a minute to do, and the entire sequence for that target area should take no more than five minutes.

- These are exercises that tone and sculpt to give you a dancer's body. You don't need the skills of a dancer to learn how to exercise like one!

- You can do these exercises every day if you choose to, and can work up to incorporating a towel or hand weights as you see fit. I recommend hand weights between three and eight pounds. Always start with the very lightest weight and work your way up.

- Many of the exercises—especially those for the arms, chest, and legs—can be done when you're taking a break from work, in the office, or when traveling. Try to avoid making any excuses about not having time to work out—and take the workout on the go with you!

- Building on these routines will enable you to customize every workout—you can switch these sequences around in any way that you like. In the next chapter, you'll see how to build on these sequences for even more comprehensive routines.

- We all have those days! So when you are very busy, you don't have to do all these exercises at once. You can do one sequence before you leave the house for work, one or two during the day, and one or two more when you're back home. Many studies have found that you can still reap the health benefits of exercise without doing one long workout. Just keep moving!

MY FAVORITE
FIVE-MINUTE WORKOUTS

1. Target: Your Butt

The butt is a problem area for so many of us. I've been fortunate to have trained in dance for so long that my lower body gets a great workout when I'm rehearsing and performing. Whenever I have any time away from the dance floor, I like to keep focusing on my buns with this five-minute routine.

Total Time: Five minutes.

Equipment Needed: An exercise mat, towel, or soft surface.

What to Do: Perform these five exercises for one minute each.

Glute Bridge

1. Lie flat on the floor on your back with hands by your sides and your knees bent. Your feet should be shoulder-width apart.

2. Pushing mainly with your heels, lift your hips off the floor while keeping your back straight.

3. Squeeze your glutes at the top.

4. Slowly go back to the starting position, then repeat for thirty seconds.

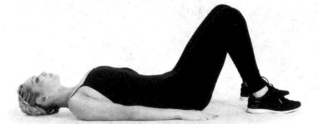

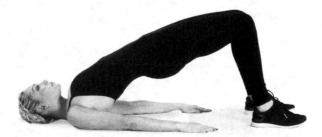

Straight-Leg Lifts on All Fours

1. Position yourself on all fours with your shoulders over your wrists and your hips over your knees.

2. Extend one leg straight behind with your toe on the floor.

3. Keeping your leg straight and toes pointed, lift your leg to hip height and slowly lower.

4. Repeat for thirty seconds.

5. Switch sides and repeat the movement for thirty seconds.

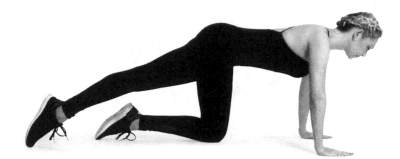

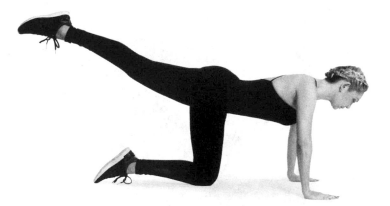

Crossovers on All Fours

1. Position yourself on all fours with your shoulders over your wrists and your hips over your knees.

2. Do this three-part movement:

   A. Lift your right knee off the floor and press your right heel up toward the ceiling.

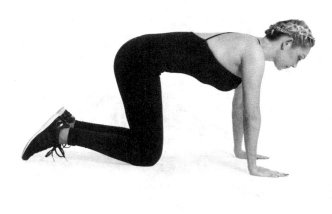

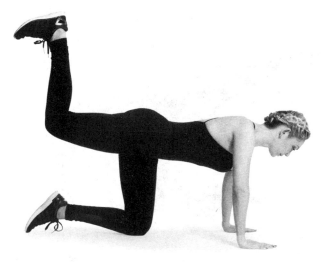

    B. Cross your right knee behind your left leg.

    C. Lift your heel back toward the ceiling and lower it.

3. Repeat for thirty seconds.

4. Switch sides and repeat the movement with the opposite leg for thirty seconds.

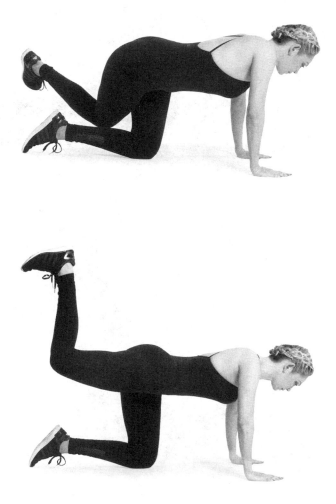

Side-Lying Leg Lifts

1. Lie on your left side with your head on your left arm, with both legs extended straight out.

2. Keeping your feet flexed, lift and slowly lower your top leg.

3. Repeat for thirty seconds.

4. Switch sides and repeat for thirty seconds.

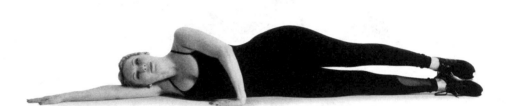

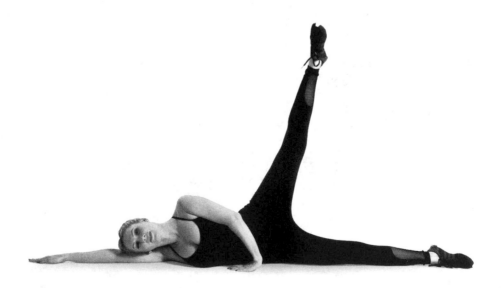

Side-Lying Clams

1. Lie on your left side with your head on your left arm.

2. Keeping both legs together, flex your hips to forty-five degrees and bend your knees to approximately ninety degrees.

3. Keep your feet touching while you open your right leg toward the ceiling, then lower it back down slowly until your knees touch.

4. Repeat for thirty seconds.

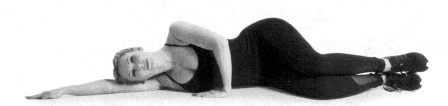

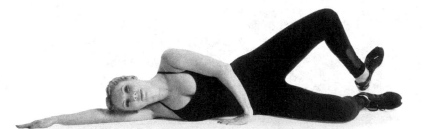

2. Target: Your Chest and Arms

When I work out my upper body I don't want to become too bulky. I balance these exercises to maintain a toned, sculpted look.

Total Time: Five minutes.

Equipment Needed: An exercise mat, towel, or soft surface; a towel for your hands or a light set of hand weights. I like to do these with a five-pound weight, but you can choose anywhere from three to eight pounds. Do what feels right for that day's workout!

What to Do: Perform these five exercises for one minute each.

Push-up

1. Start in a High Plank (page 170) position with your shoulders over your wrists. Maintain a straight line from your head to your toes.

2. Lower yourself downward until your chest almost touches the floor as you inhale.

3. Breathe out, and press your body back up to the starting position.

4. Do as many as you can in one minute. Form matters more than speed!

TIP
Newbies to the Push-up or those with any lower back issues can start out with a Half Push-up. Let your knees stay on the floor and focus on keeping your chest lifted throughout the push-yourself-up movement.

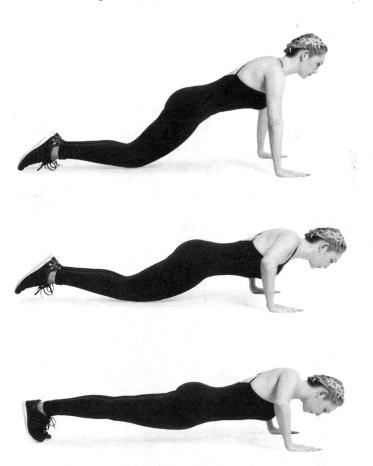

Bicep Curl

1. Grab the towel or hand weights with both hands, palms facing toward your body.

2. Balance on one leg and place the towel under the knee of your lifted leg.

3. Bend at the elbows and bring your hands toward your shoulders.

4. Repeat for thirty seconds.

5. Switch legs and repeat for thirty more seconds.

TIP
If you're using hand weights, lift one knee to hip height while you perform the curls.

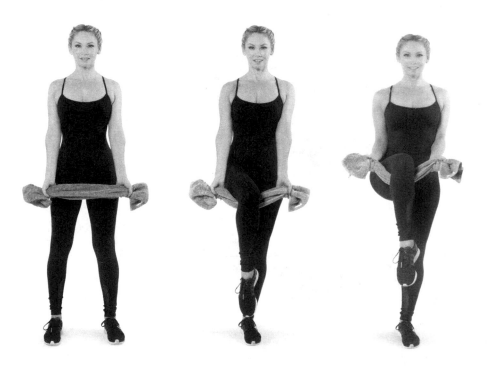

Triceps Dip

1. Sit on the floor with your feet hip-width apart and knees bent. Place your arms behind your hips, your hands on the floor, and your fingers facing your body.

2. Raise your hips off the floor.

3. Bend your elbows and lower your hips toward the floor, then extend your arms and squeeze the backs of your upper arms together.

TIP
A small bend will make a big difference here. The stronger you get, the lower you'll be able to bring your hips to the ground.

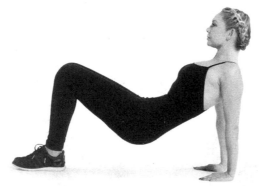

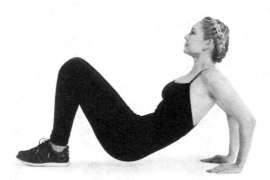

Chest Scoop

1. Start standing with your feet hip-width apart.

2. Grab the towel with your arms held out wider than your hips and your palms facing away from your body.

3. Create tension on the towel by pulling it taut and raise your arms to shoulder height. Hold the position for one minute.

4. Maintain the tension on the towel, holding it strongly in front of you as you lower your arms.

TIP
If you feel like you're straining by holding this position for a minute, hold it for ten to twenty seconds and repeat the motion several times.

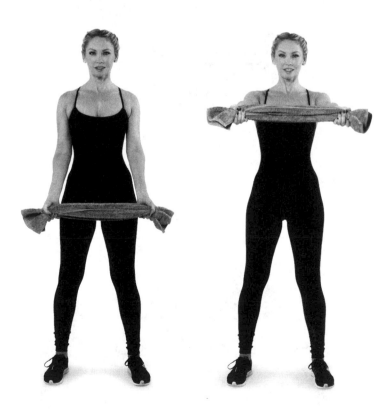

Side-Lying Triceps

1. Lie on your left side in a fetal position, with your knees bent to a forty-five-degree angle, left arm wrapped across your chest, right hand flat on the floor in front of your left arm.

2. By pressing your hand into the floor, raise your head and shoulders off of the floor and flex the back of your upper arm at the top.

3. Continue moving up and down for one minute.

TIP
Avoid locking your elbows. You can keep your chest and shoulders engaged by bending your elbows slightly. If you feel like you're straining, then make the movement smaller.

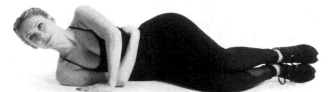

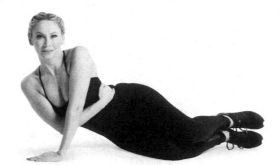

The shoulders and back are often neglected, but these are large foundational muscle groups. When I'm dancing, my partners always comment on how challenging it is to stay in a dancer's hold. By combining the exercises here you'll work all the muscles required to maintain that position.

Total Time: Five minutes.

Equipment Needed: An exercise mat, towel, or soft surface; a towel for your hands or a light set of hand weights.

What to Do: Perform these five exercises for one minute each.

Bent-Over Row

1. Grab the towel with both hands, palms facing away from your body.

2. Position yourself by bending your knees and pushing your hips back so you are slightly bent over.

3. Contract your abs and pull the towel up toward your sides, squeezing your back muscles. Have your elbows graze your rib cage.

4. Hold for one second, then lower your arms back to the starting position. Repeat the pulling movement.

TIP
If you're using hand weights, be sure to control the weights on the way down.

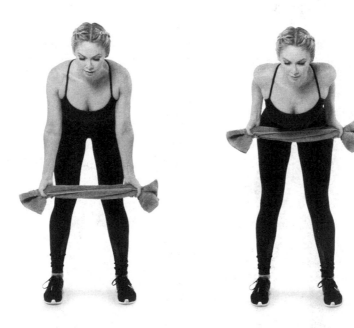

Shoulder Press

1. Start standing with your feet hip-width apart.

2. Grab the towel with your hands outstretched in front of your shoulders at chest height.

3. Create tension on the towel by pulling it taut, and press your arms overhead.

4. Maintain the tension and lower your arms back to chest height.

TIP
If you're using hand weights, control them. Avoid shrugging your shoulders up so you maintain the space between your shoulders and your ears.

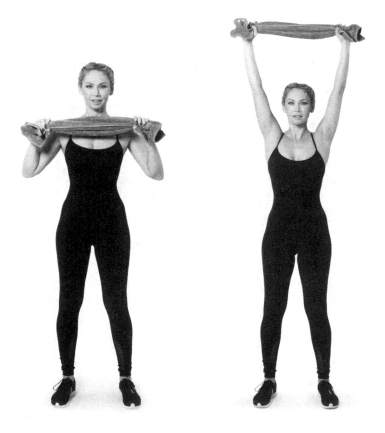

Front Raise

1. Start standing with your feet hip-width apart.

2. Grab the towel with your arms at hip width and palms facing toward your body.

3. Create tension on the towel by pulling it taut, and raise your arms to shoulder height.

4. Maintain the tension and lower your arms back to hip height.

TIP
If you're using hand weights, try to keep your wrists flat throughout the exercise, avoiding rotation.

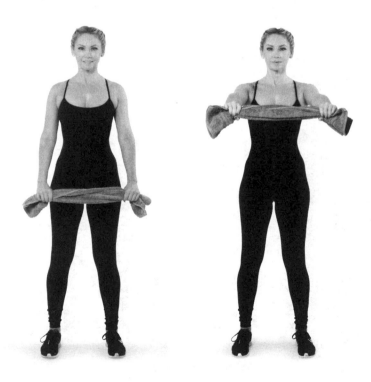

Bent-Over Fly

1. From a standing position, bend your knees slightly and push your hips back so you're bent over with a flat back.

2. Let your arms fall toward the floor, palms facing in.

3. Keep the arms straight as you raise them up to your sides, to shoulder height.

4. Squeeze your shoulder blades together at the top, then slowly lower arms down. Repeat movement.

TIP
If you're using hand weights, be sure to keep a slight bend in your elbows.

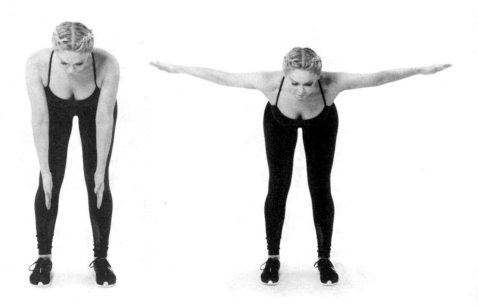

Shoulder Retractions

1. Start standing with your feet hip-width apart, arms bent at your sides, palms facing up.

2. Keeping your elbows glued to your sides, open your arms as if you are flashing someone (not that you would . . . but if you did!).

3. Squeeze your shoulder blades together, then return your arms to the starting position. Repeat the movement.

TIP
If you're using hand weights, keep your elbows in position while maintaining a straight wrist.

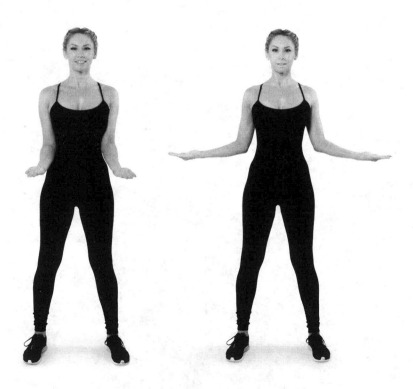

4. Target: Your Legs

I've incorporated some of my favorite movements here to give you a true dancer's lower-body workout. You'll tone and sculpt your legs using your own body weight in a series of lunges and squats.

Total Time: Five minutes.

Equipment Needed: None.

What to Do: Perform these five exercises for one minute each.

Wall Sit

1. Stand with your back flat against a wall.

2. Walk your feet about two feet in front of you, spread about six inches apart.

3. Slide your back down the wall, bending your knees until they are at about a ninety-degree angle.

4. Hold this position.

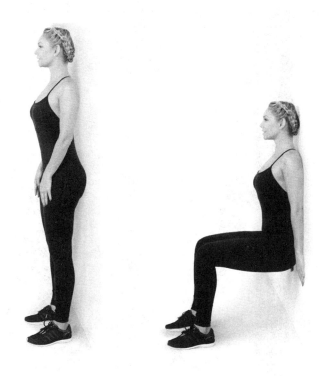

Paso Lunge + Cape Arms

1. Start standing with your feet hip-width apart.

2. Step your right leg forward across your left and bend your knees, lowering your hips toward the ground.

3. As you lower yourself down, cross your right arm in the direction you are stepping. Imagine you are swinging a cape.

4. Repeat for thirty seconds.

5. Switch legs and repeat for thirty more seconds.

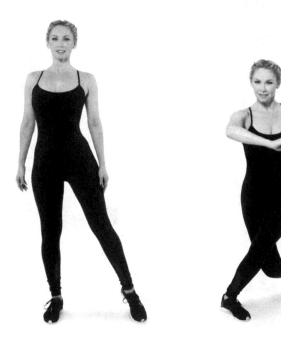

Plié + Calf Raise

1. Stand with your feet wider than hip-width apart, toes turned out, and hands on your hips.

2. Bend your knees over your toes and lower yourself slowly down until you feel tension.

3. Extend your knees and rise out of the lowered position. When you get back to the starting position, raise your heels so you're on your tiptoes.

4. Repeat by lowering into the Plié and raising into the Calf Raise on tiptoe for one minute.

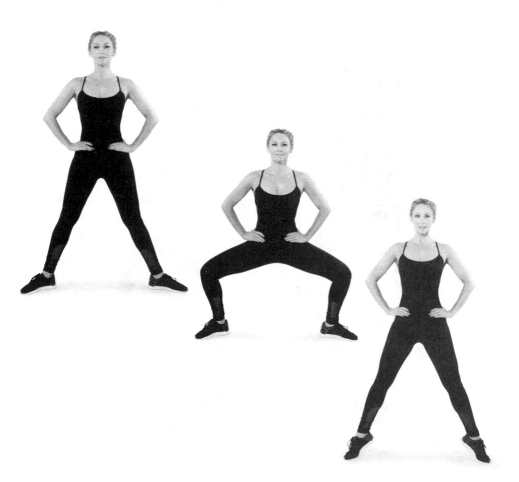

Curtsy Lunges

1. Stand with your feet wider than hip-width apart.

2. Step your left leg behind your right so your thighs cross, bending both knees as if you were curtsying.

3. Return to the standing position and switch sides. Continue the curtsy movement from side to side.

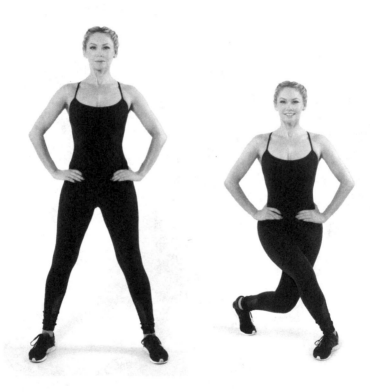

Squat + Arabesque

1. Stand with feet shoulder width apart.

2. Bend your knees, lowering your hips toward the ground.

3. As you straighten one leg, raise the other up behind you while simultaneously reaching your arms forward.

4. Alternate sides.

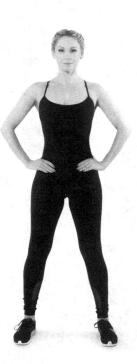

5. Target: Cardio

I love to mix some cardio into each of my workouts. Whether I'm warming up or going for a jog, cardio helps get my heart pumping and makes me sweat. You'll learn a bit more about the benefits of cardio and how you can incorporate it into your workouts in the next chapter, but for now, let's get started with this straight-forward five-minute cardio routine.

Total Time: Five minutes.

Equipment Needed: An exercise mat, towel, or soft surface; supportive, comfortable exercise shoes.

What to Do: Perform these five exercises for one minute each.

High-Knee Run on Spot

1. Start standing with your legs shoulder width apart. Your arms should be bent at your sides.

2. Stay in the same spot and lift your right knee and then your left knee at a running pace.

3. Swing your arms as if you were jogging.

TIP
If you have knee issues, you can march in place rather than run in place.

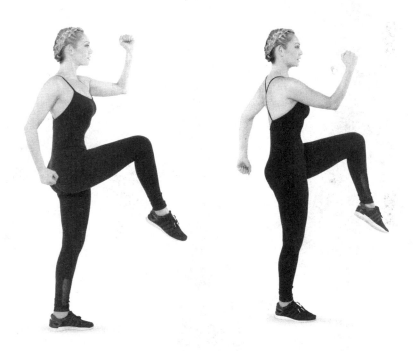

Plié Pulse + Jump

1. Start standing with your legs hip-width apart, toes facing out at a forty-five-degree angle.

2. Lower your hips down to about knee height and do three small pulses, then explode up off your toes in a jump and click your heels together.

TIPS
- To soften the landing, bend your knees as your feet come back in contact with the floor.

- If you have knee issues, omit the jump and simply rise up onto your toes.

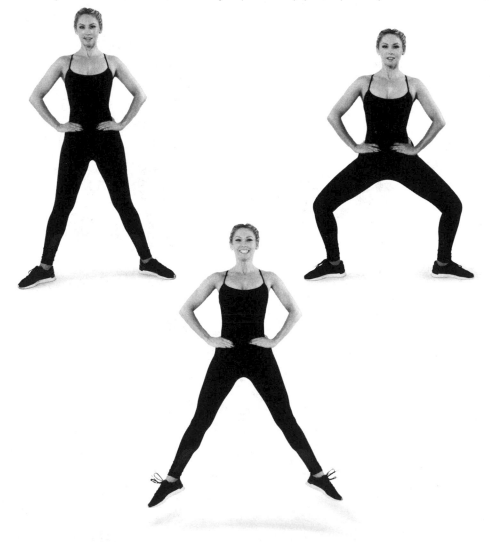

Burpees

1. Start standing tall, then squat down and place your hands on the floor in front of you.

2. Jump your legs out behind you so that you are in a High Plank(page 170) position, then jump them back into a crouched position.

3. Jump up as high as possible and reach up with your arms.

TIP
Try to do these with increasing speed once you master the move.

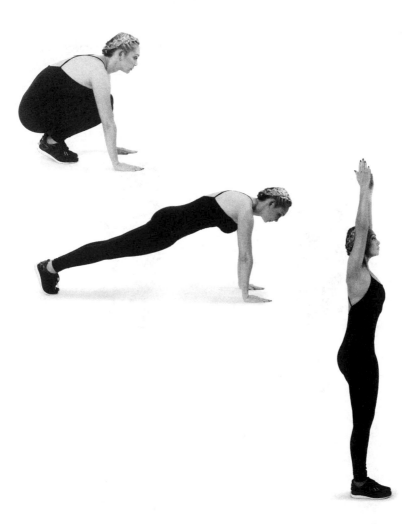

Single-Leg Knee Drives

1. Start standing with one leg behind the other.

2. Bend your front knee about six inches, then hinge forward from the hips while reaching your arms forward one at a time.

3. Maintain the bend in your front knee and the hinge from the hips as you pull your back knee in toward your chest while pulling your arms in.

4. Repeat the knee pull for thirty seconds.

5. Switch sides halfway and repeat for thirty seconds.

TIP
For more of a challenge, pick up the pace and get lower on your front leg.

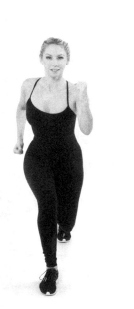 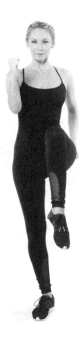

Crossover Jumping Jacks

1. Start standing with your feet together.

2. Jump your legs apart and reach your arms straight out to shoulder height, palms facing up.

3. Jump your feet back together, crossing your right leg in front of your left leg and your right arm in front of your left arm in front of your chest.

4. Switch sides.

5. Repeat jumping, alternating your leg and arm crossing in front.

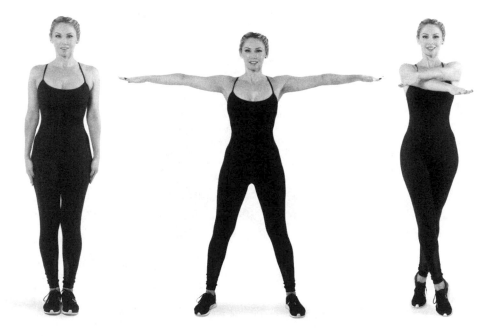

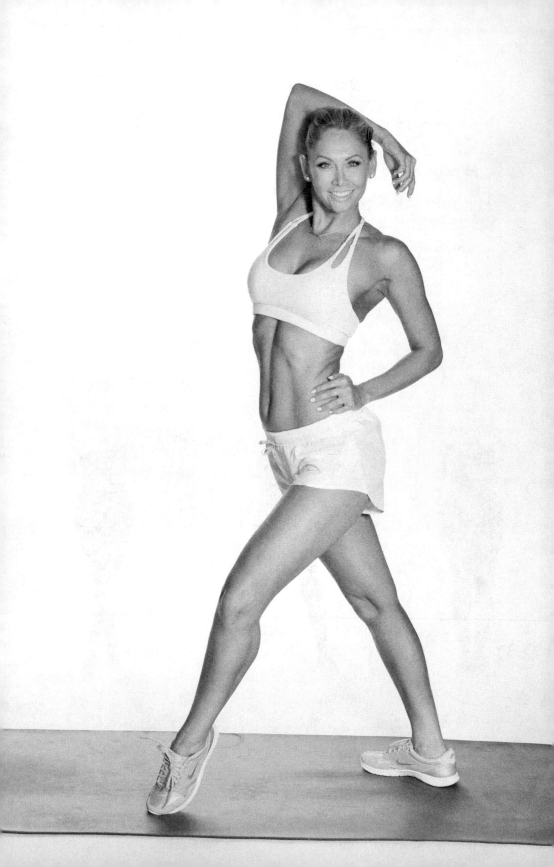

9

Total-Body Workouts

As a dancer it's important to keep your entire body strong. I like to combine the routines we have worked on so far to create a total-body workout. By completing these total-body workouts you're creating more lean muscle mass. This leads to burning more calories, even at rest.

You can perform all of the workouts here with your own body weight, a jump rope, and a towel or a set of hand weights. There are six total-body workouts to add some variety to your routine. Keep these tips in mind:

- Before each workout, do a warm-up for one to three minutes. I like to jump rope. Other options: jog lightly in place, march in place, or just walk to get your heart rate going.

- Next, do a core workout from chapter 7 to engage the core and complete the warm-up.

- Follow this with one of the circuits below. They all use different exercises from chapter 8.

TOTAL-BODY WORKOUT #1

Here, I've created two circuits that each have three exercises. You'll be working your upper body, lower body, and cardiovascular system with this dynamic routine.

Equipment Needed: An exercise mat, towel, or soft surface; a towel or set of light hand weights for the bicep curls.

What to Do: Perform each exercise for twenty repetitions. Complete two sets of each circuit.

Circuit 1	Plié + Calf Raise Push-up High-Knee Run on Spot
Circuit 2	Bicep Curl Glute Bridge Bicycle Crunch

TOTAL-BODY WORKOUT #2

I've broken this workout into three circuits of three exercises each. You'll master the movements on your first two rounds and have the chance to really push yourself on round three.

Equipment Needed: An exercise mat, towel, or soft surface; a towel or set of light hand weights.

What to Do: Perform each exercise for twelve repetitions. Complete three sets of each circuit.

Circuit 1	Squat + Arabesque Shoulder Press
Circuit 2	Bent-Over Row Burpees
Circuit 3	Latin Hip Rolls Plank Cinch

TOTAL-BODY WORKOUT #3

One of my personal favorites! This is the ultimate endurance workout. I've combined eight exercises back-to-back that will push you to the limit.

Equipment Needed: An exercise mat, towel, or soft surface.

What to Do: Perform two sets of all eight exercises.

For set one, do sixteen repetitions of each exercise.

For set two, do twelve repetitions of each exercise.

Plié Pulse + Jump
Paso Lunge + Cape Arms, Right Side
Paso Lunge + Cape Arms, Left Side
Triceps Dip
Salsa Combo Twist
Side-Lying Leg Lifts, Right Side
Side-Lying Leg Lifts, Left Side
Back Extensions

TOTAL-BODY WORKOUT #4

This is an interval-style circuit workout. You'll be jumping for joy with the Jacks in circuit 1, but your glutes will be on fire by the time you hit the Clams in circuit 2.

Equipment Needed: An exercise mat, towel, or soft surface; a towel or set of light hand weights.

What to Do: Perform each exercise for forty-five seconds. Take a fifteen-to-thirty-second rest between exercises. Complete two sets of each circuit.

Circuit 1	Wall Sit Chest Scoop Crossover Jumping Jacks
Circuit 2	Shoulder Retractions Side-Lying Clams, Right Side-Lying Clams, Left

TOTAL-BODY WORKOUT #5

This a time-based workout. The goal is to keep a steady pace while maintaining proper form.

Equipment Needed: An exercise mat, towel, or soft surface; a towel or set of light hand weights.

What to Do: Perform each exercise for thirty seconds. Take a fifteen-to-thirty-second rest between exercises. Complete three sets of each circuit.

Circuit 1	Jive Crunch, Right Side Jive Crunch, Left Side
Circuit 2	Bent-Over Fly High Plank + Oblique Knee Pulls
Circuit 3	Crossovers on All Fours, Right Crossovers on All Fours, Left

TOTAL-BODY WORKOUT #6

My go-to interval routine using my favorite workout accessory—the jump rope! You'll alternate between strength exercises and jumping rope, achieving a total-body burn.

Equipment Needed: An exercise mat, towel, or soft surface; a towel or set of light hand weights; a jump rope.

What to Do: Perform one minute of each exercise for one set. Take a fifteen-to-thirty-second rest between exercises. To modify, only jump rope for twenty seconds.

Curtsy Lunges
Jump Rope
Front Raise
Jump Rope
Waistline Reach
Jump Rope
Side-Lying Triceps, Right
Side-Lying Triceps, Left
Jump Rope
Straight-Leg Lifts on All Fours, Right Side
Straight-Leg Lifts on All Fours, Left Side
Jump Rope
Basic Crunch
Jump Rope

Let's Talk About Cardio!

When I'm dancing, it's usually in one-and-a-half-to-two-minute bursts. It's so challenging to get through a rehearsal because you're taxing your body over and over again to get the routine right.

In order to maintain that pace I like to do a mix of interval training and cardio exercise. Cardio is a very important part of achieving a dancer's body and supporting your complete workout. I like to do at least fifteen minutes of cardio along with the targeted exercises from chapter 8. When I have time, I even try to incorporate some cardio in addition to the total-body workouts from this chapter. Doing both—cardio to strengthen your heart and lungs, and toning to strengthen your muscles—is the ideal workout for total-body fitness. You can't really have one without the other!

Cardio, which is short for cardiovascular exercise, is any kind of movement that gets your heart rate up. This not only strengthens your heart, it improves how your body intakes and uses oxygen. In addition, during cardio exercise you are moving large muscle groups in your arms, legs, and hips, which burns mega-calories.

Cardio exercise is absolutely essential for anyone who wants optimal health. Here's why:

- Cardio helps you feel energized and confident. The more you do, the more energy you have.

- Cardio also lowers your resting heart rate. A lower resting heart rate means that your everyday activities will seem easier over time, as you'll have more stamina.

- Cardio reduces stress by increasing the production of your brain's feel-good neurotransmitters, known as endorphins. This can give you a wonderful flooding rush of happiness during a workout or afterward.

- Cardio can help lower anxiety and depression.

- Cardio also reduces stress by helping you focus and concentrate on your physical movement. I always find that exercise helps clear my head when something's bothering me. I love to turn up the music and just let loose for a while!

- Cardio is great for your brain. It can preserve and improve learning and memory; your brain is always making new connections (this is called plasticity), and exercise helps stimulate these connections, no matter how old you are. Learning new steps during a dance or exercise class is a particularly good way to wake up your brain.

- Cardio is one of the cheapest ways to take care of your health! It has been proven to reduce the risk of heart disease and some types of cancer, obesity, high blood pressure, and type 2 diabetes.

- Cardio helps you sleep better and more profoundly. Just don't go for a long workout right before bed, as you'll be so energized you might have trouble shutting your eyes!

- Cardio is great for your skin. It improves your blood flow, making your skin positively glow. (Just be sure to use sunscreen when you work out outdoors, please, no matter what your skin tone.)

- Cardio helps to strengthen your immune system. This may leave you less susceptible to catching colds, bugs that might be going around, or the seasonal flu.

Well, I don't know about you, but I'm convinced! Here are my favorite types of cardio exercises:

Walking: One of my favorite things to do is walk my puppy, Lola. I make our walks more cardio-intense when I alternate between a power walk and my normal pace. If you are at the gym, set the treadmill on a 1.0 incline or higher, and put on some music to keep you on the beat and going strong. Try to walk for thirty to sixty minutes. A great way to do interval training is to raise and lower the incline along with your speed. If you're just walking outside, try to alternate your playlist between fast and slow songs so you get motivated to speed up with the upbeat tempo.

Hiking: I love hiking. There's always something new to see and the time goes by so quickly—it really doesn't seem like "exercise." Take a friend and go exploring!

Biking: If you have a bike path in your area, get outside and cruise, but don't forget your helmet! If you don't have a nearby path or if the weather isn't cooperating, most gyms offer two types of exercise bikes: upright and recumbent. If you have any lower-back issues, stick to the recumbent bike, as it puts less stress on that area. Try to ride for thirty to sixty minutes. As with the treadmill, try to vary your speed and the resistance to make your workout more interesting.

Swimming: Whether it's at the beach, in a lake, or in a pool, swimming can be very therapeutic. It's also great for creating long, lean muscles without placing any stress on your joints. Try to swim for thirty to sixty minutes. You can also try walking or jogging in the water, as the extra resistance of pushing against the water gives you a high-intensity workout.

If you're finding yourself short on time there are many opportunities for cardiovascular movement throughout the day that you might be missing. Here are simple ways you can stay fit without even realizing you're working out:

- Take the stairs.

- Walk around the house or even march in place while you're on the phone.

- Park far away from the grocery store.

- Do some salsa arms in your chair at work (you know you've always wanted to!).

- March on the spot when you're in line for coffee.

- Do squats or pliés while you're brushing your teeth.

Don't Forget to Warm Up First—and Stretch Afterward

People sometimes think that they should stretch before they work out, but that's a misconception. You should only stretch after your exercises. The reason for this is that if you start stretching cold, you're more likely to pull a muscle.

That being said, you definitely need to warm up before you get moving, especially when you're planning your cardio sessions.

Over the years, I've found that the best way to warm up is with a little bit of cardio as well as a core workout. When I was on tour I'd jump rope for a few minutes, then gather some friends for a session of core exercises. We would do a combination of planks, crunches, and back extensions just like the routines in chapter 7. By focusing on the workout, we were not only engaging our cores but concentrating on our breathing— and getting ourselves into the right mind-set for performing.

Even if you're not a dancer, add a bit of a warm-up before you do any cardio workouts. If you like to jog, then walk for a few minutes first. If you like to go to a gym, walk from your car or do a few minutes of walking on a treadmill or a slow ride on a bicycle. This will get your heart pumping and the blood flowing to your muscles, which will help prevent injuries.

Then, when your workout is done, it's time to stretch. Your muscles will be warm and will appreciate the attention!

Workout #1: Restorative on page 230 in the next chapter contains several of my favorite stretches. These are the ones you should do:

- Chest Opener to Upper-Back Release

- Neck Stretch

- Lying Hamstring Stretch

- Spinal Rotation

- Figure 4

After a tough show or rehearsal I love to use a foam roller or tennis ball to support my stretching. If you've got a very tight knot you can even use a golf ball—but be warned, it might make you wince a little bit. Keep at it, because it's helping to break up the muscle soreness and you'll feel so much better afterward. This technique is called "myofascial release." It's used to help treat and prevent muscle soreness through gently applying sustained pressure to affected areas, which include not only your muscles but your fascia—the connective tissue supporting your joints and muscles. (Any knots you feel are actually gnarled-up fascia.) Place a tennis ball or foam roller under any part of your body that may be tender. While taking full inhales and exhales, slowly roll that area over the ball/foam roller. Keep rolling that area for ninety seconds to up to three minutes before moving to the next spot.

MONDAY	TUESDAY	WEDNESDAY	THURSDAY
1 Workout 1	**2** Workout 2	**3** Rest	**4** Workout 3
8 Workout 5	**9** Workout 6	**10** Rest	**11** Workout 1
15 Rest	**16** Workout 4	**17** Workout 5	**18** Cardio
22 Rest	**23** Workout 3	**24** Workout 4	**25** Workout 5
29 Workout 2 (Option to add Workout 5)	**30** Workout 3 (Option to add Workout 6)		

The next time you're sitting in front of the TV, reading a book, or going online, remind yourself to stretch. Hop down onto the floor and enjoy your downtime while helping your body recover!

Thirty-Day Total-Body Workout Calendar

Here is a suggested calendar so you can optimize your thirty-day fitness program. This calendar will help you plan your total-body workouts with the cardio component added. As you know, some of my favorite cardio workouts are walking, hiking, biking, swimming, and, of course, dancing!

FRIDAY	SATURDAY	SUNDAY
5 Cardio	**6** Rest	**7** Workout 4
12 Cardio	**13** Workout 2	**14** Workout 3
19 Workout 6	**20** Workout 1	**21** Workout 2
26 Cardio	**27** Workout 6	**28** Workout 1 (Option to add Workout 4)

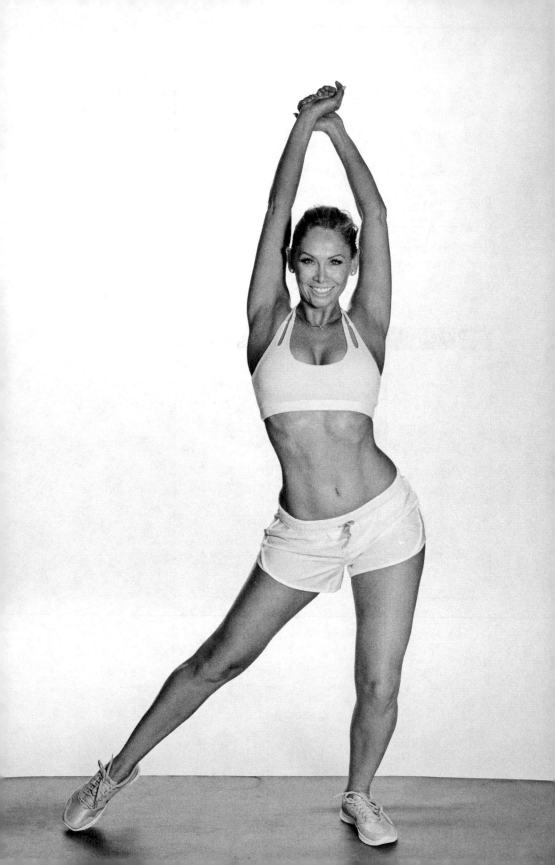

10

Specialty Workouts

Sometimes I want to mix up my routine and try something completely out of the box. These specialty workouts will take between fifteen and twenty minutes and can be done absolutely anywhere—in a hotel room when you're traveling, outside at the park, at the gym, at home, wherever you like. By switching up the exercises and locations, you'll keep things fresh and stay motivated to stick with your program.

Workout #1: Restorative

This is a great workout to do when you feel the need to move but you don't want to overdo it. It is very effective to help you achieve a sense of calm. You'll feel strong and relaxed after completing these postures. And you can use the stretches after any workout to help you cool down and release any tight muscles.

Equipment Needed: An exercise mat, towel, or soft surface; a towel.

What to Do: Make a playlist of a few songs, about twenty minutes in length, that you know are relaxing, rather than super-stimulating. Perform each exercise for the specified time or repetitions.

Relevé

1. Start standing with your feet in first position (heels together, toes facing out).

2. Slowly lift your heels off the ground and then lower them.

3. Repeat sixteen times.

TIP
Small movements make a big difference! Each time you perform this exercise you'll be able to lift your heels a bit higher off the ground.

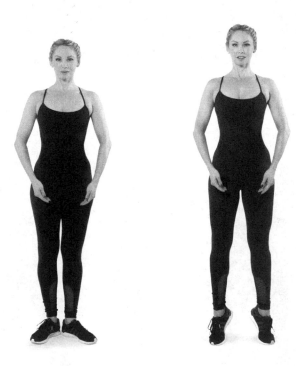

Chest Opener to Upper-Back Release

1. Start standing with your feet shoulder-width apart.
2. Open your arms to shoulder height with your elbows bent at a ninety-degree angle, palms open and facing forward. That movement is a chest stretch.
3. Next, close your hands together in front of you and clasp them together, flip the palms away from your body, and push your hands away, allowing your neck to release to your chest and your shoulder blades to move apart.
4. Repeat eight times.

TIP
You want to feel this release in your upper back.

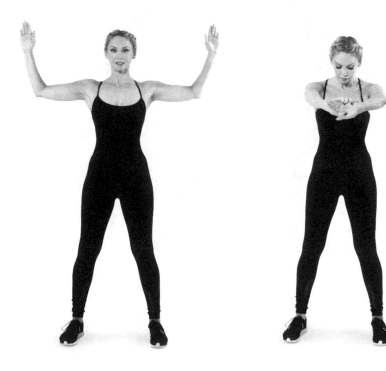

Neck Stretch

1. Start standing with your feet shoulder width apart.
2. Reach behind your back and grab your left wrist with your right hand, then pull your wrist toward your right hip as you drop your head to your right shoulder.
3. Hold this stretch for four counts of eight, or approximately thirty seconds.
4. Repeat on the left side.

TIP
You should feel a stretch down the sides of your neck and the front of your shoulders.

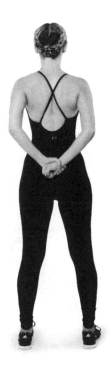
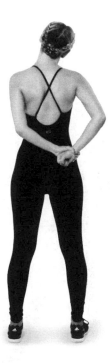

Lateral Lunges

1. Start standing with your feet wider than hip-width apart, hands on your hips.

2. Hinge forward slightly from the hips and lean onto one leg, bending your knee about six inches.

3. Shift from side to side.

4. Repeat for eight counts of eight, or approximately one minute.

TIP
When you're shifting your weight, you should feel the stretch in your inner thigh.

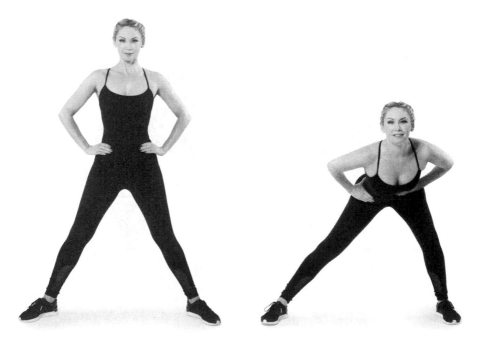

Hip Flexor Lunge

1. Start standing with your feet hip-width apart.

2. Step your left foot forward about two feet. Only step forward as much as you can while keeping the heel of your right foot on the floor.

3. Reach your arms up and slightly lean back until you feel a stretch in the front of your right hip.

4. Hold this pose for a count of four.

5. Repeat the above steps on the other side.

6. Repeat for eight counts of eight, or approximately one minute.

TIP
If looking up toward the ceiling makes you feel dizzy, then look straight ahead.

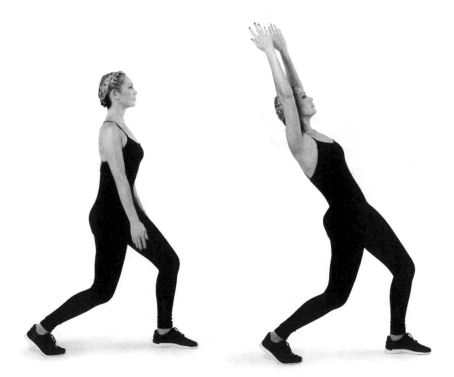

Lying Hamstring Stretch

1. Lie flat on your back.

2. Lift your right leg off the floor and wrap a towel around your foot.

3. Slowly extend your knee to the point of mild tension, not pain.

4. Hold the stretch for one minute.

5. Repeat with your left leg.

TIP
You should feel this stretch all the way from your calves to your hamstrings to your glutes.

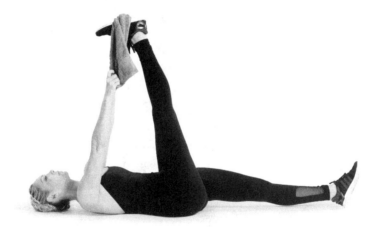

Spinal Rotation

1. Lie flat on your back, with your arms out to the sides, palms pressing into the ground.

2. Lift your right knee toward your chest and wrap your left hand over your knee. Slowly rotate your knee across your body to the point of mild tension, not pain.

3. Hold the twist for one minute.

4. Repeat on your left side.

TIP
To increase the intensity of the pose, turn your head in the direction of the stretch, on each side.

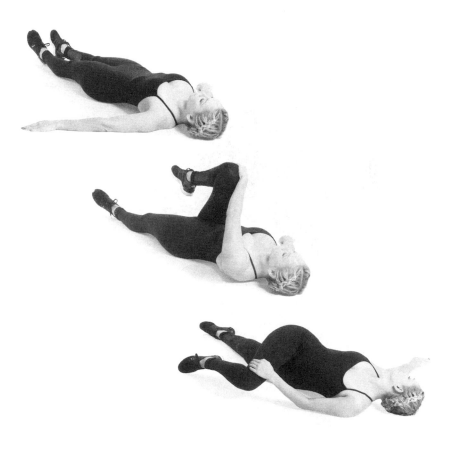

Figure 4

1. Lie flat on your back.

2. Lift your right leg off the ground and bend your knee so it's positioned above your hip.

3. Cross your left leg over the right.

4. Reach your hands through to your right leg. Grab on to it and slowly pull it in toward your body.

5. Hold the stretch for one minute.

6. Repeat with your left leg.

TIP
You should feel this stretch in your hips and glutes.

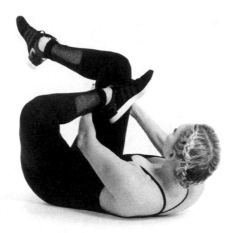

Workout #2: Chair Workout

This is a terrific workout when you're traveling, especially if you're in a hotel room or at a friend's house and don't have much time or access to a gym. Since I travel so much, I always try to do this routine when I know there will be jet lag due to all the time changes—it really does help you adjust, and makes you feel energized and refreshed.

Equipment Needed: A sturdy chair (not on wheels!). You will use the chair only for balance and support.

What to Do: Imagine the chair is your ballet barre, and use it for support. Perform each exercise for the specified time or repetitions. Complete all six exercises and then repeat the entire sequence a second time.

Plié to Relevé

1. Start standing behind your chair with your hands placed lightly on the top.

2. Place your feet slightly wider than hip-width apart.

3. Bend your knees, lowering your hips toward the ground into a plié position.

4. Extend your knees and raise your body back up.

5. At the top of the movement, lift your heels off the ground into a relevé position.

6. Repeat for one minute.

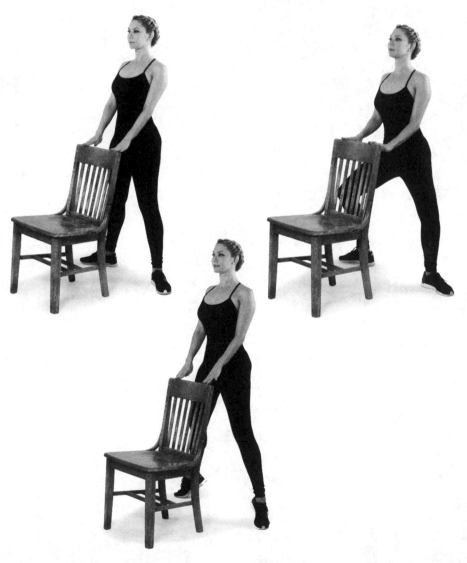

Arabesque Lifts

1. Start standing behind your chair with your hands placed lightly on the top.

2. Place your left leg behind your right, and slightly bend your right leg.

3. Point your left toes, then lift and lower your left leg. Be sure to squeeze your left glutes at the top of the movement.

4. Repeat for one minute.

5. Repeat with your right leg.

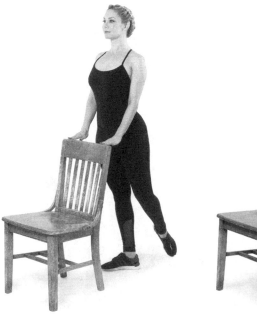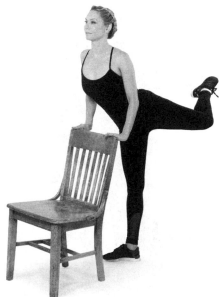

Parallel Plié Pulses

1. Start standing behind your chair with your hands placed lightly on the top.

2. Place your feet at hip width, toes facing forward.

3. Bend your knees, lowering your hips toward the ground until your hips are in line with your knees.

4. Holding that position, perform small pulses up and down.

5. Continue the pulses for one minute.

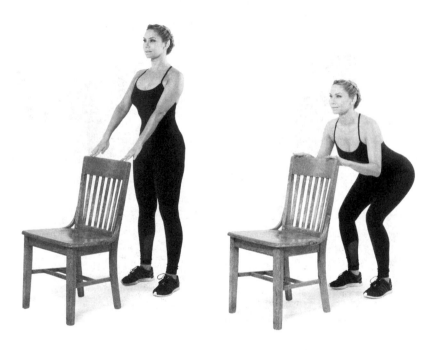

Curtsy + Oblique Knee Lifts

1. Start standing to the left side of your chair with your right hand placed lightly on top for balance and your left hand behind your head.

2. Step your left foot behind your right, lowering your hips into a curtsy position.

3. As you rise back to standing, lift your left knee up to the side, bringing your knee to your left elbow.

4. Repeat for one minute.

5. Repeat with your right leg.

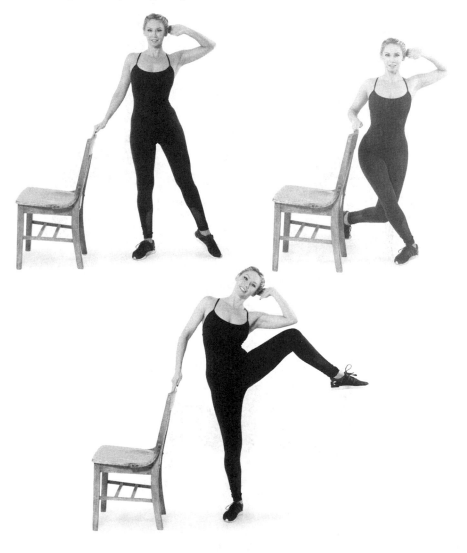

Triceps Dips

1. Sit in the chair, holding on to the edge with both hands.

2. Slide your bottom off the seat and hold yourself up with your arms straight.

3. Slowly lower your body as you bend your elbows, then straighten your arms.

4. Repeat sixteen times.

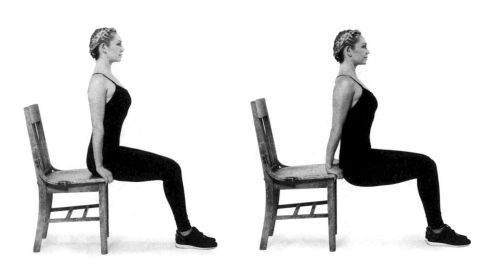

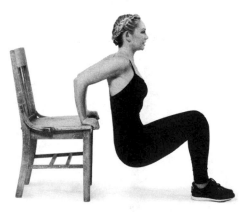

Hover Squats

1. Start standing about six inches in front of your chair.

2. Extend your arms in front at chest height.

3. Slowly lower your bottom and stop right before you tap the chair.

4. Hold the hover for approximately ten seconds.

5. Repeat ten times.

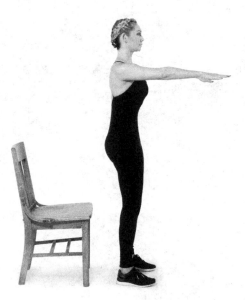

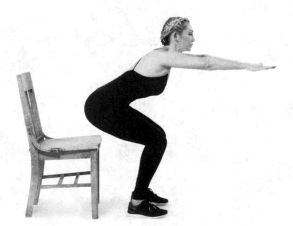

Workout #3: Slider Workout

If you're looking to take your workout to the next level, the slider challenge is for you! This routine will help you improve your balance and lower-body strength. If you have knee or ankle injuries, though, this may not be the workout for you!

Equipment Needed: An exercise mat and a towel. If you're exercising on a hard surface, use a towel to support this workout. If you're on a carpet, use a paper plate, as that will enable you to slide.

What to Do: Perform each exercise for the specified time or repetitions. Complete all five exercises and then repeat the entire sequence.

Squat Slide

1. Start standing with your feet shoulder-width apart and the towel under your right foot.

2. As you bend your left knee and lower your hips toward the ground, simultaneously extend your right knee and slide the towel out to the side.

3. Return to standing.

4. Switch sides.

5. Repeat for one minute on each side.

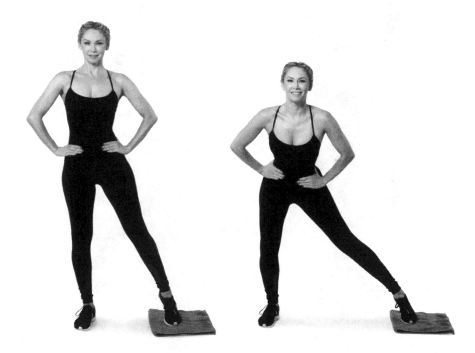

Curtsy Lunge

1. Stand with your feet wider than hip-width apart.

2. Step your left leg on the towel behind your right so your thighs cross, one foot behind the other.

3. Bending both knees as if you were curtsying, slide the towel behind you and across your body.

4. Return to standing.

5. Repeat for one minute on each side.

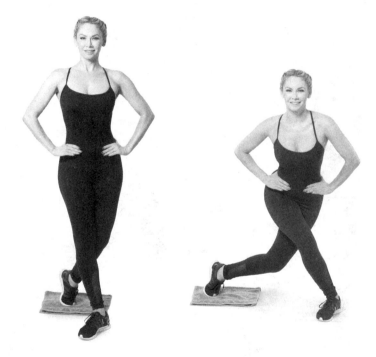

High Plank Knee Pulls

1. Place the towel under your right foot and get into the High Plank position.

2. Slide your right foot toward your chest.

3. Return your right leg back to starting position.

4. Continue sliding your foot for thirty seconds.

5. Repeat on the left side for thirty seconds.

TIP
As with the High Plank, you can modify this plank by lowering your knees to the floor.

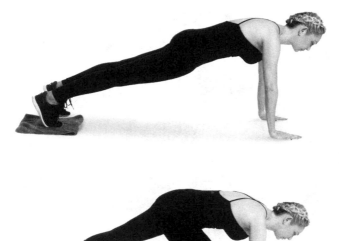

Push-Up Slides

1. Place the towel under your right hand and get into the High Plank position.

2. Lower yourself downward until your chest almost touches the floor while simultaneously extending your right arm and sliding the towel out to the side.

3. Press yourself up and return to the starting position.

4. Repeat eight times.

5. Repeat with your left arm.

TIP
This movement does not need to be big in order to be effective. A small bend of the elbow and slide of the hand strengthens your chest and arms.

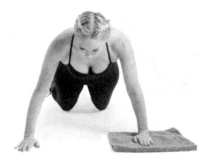

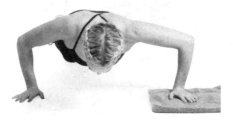

Hamstring Curls

1. Lie flat on your back with the towel under both feet.

2. Align your feet directly below your knees and press your palms into the floor with your hands by your sides.

3. Raise your hips off the floor until they are in a straight line with your knees.

4. Push your heels into the ground and drag your heels in toward your bottom.

5. Keep your hips up and continue curling for one minute.

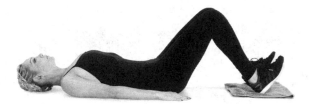

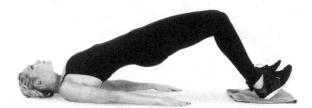

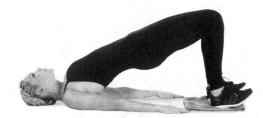

Workout #4: Partner Workout

Ballroom dancing is all about having a partner, which is why I'm partial to this routine! I also love to have someone to work out with because it makes the time fly by. Nothing is more wonderful than working hard and sharing encouragement with someone as determined as I am. (That's why these exercises are a bit more challenging than the other sequences in this chapter.) So pick your partner and let's get started!

Equipment Needed: An exercise mat, towel, or soft surface.

What to Do: Perform each exercise for one minute. Complete all five exercises and then repeat the entire sequence two more times.

Support Squats

1. Start facing away from your partner with your shoulders, lower back, and buttocks pressing against each other.

2. Bending your knees, slowly lower your hips down until they are in line with your knees.

3. Press through your feet and into your partner and return to standing.

4. Repeat for one minute.

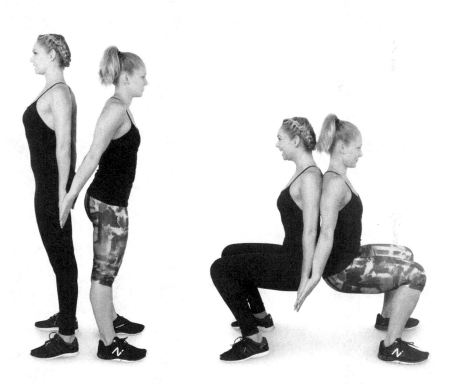

Clapping Push-up

1. Start in a High Plank position, head to head.

2. Both partners lower down into a push-up position at the same time.

3. As you return to the starting positing, lift your right hand off the floor and high-five your partner.

4. Repeat the push-up and high five with your left hand.

5. Repeat for one minute, switching hands for each push-up.

TIP
You can modify this push-up by lowering your knees to the floor.

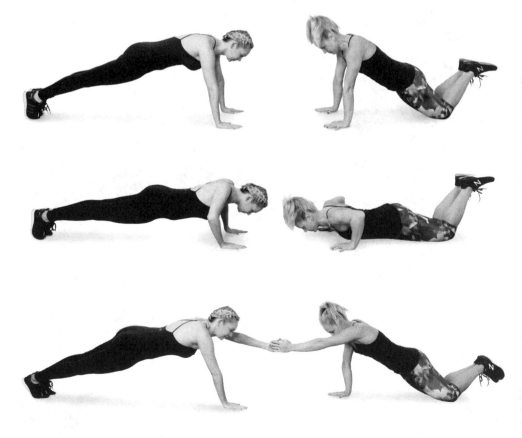

Dynamic Lunge

1. Start standing facing your partner, holding hands, with your right leg forward.

2. Bend your knees into a lunge position.

3. Jump to the same position with the left leg forward.

4. Repeat for one minute.

TIP
Use your partner to help you with balance and push you to get lower in your lunge.

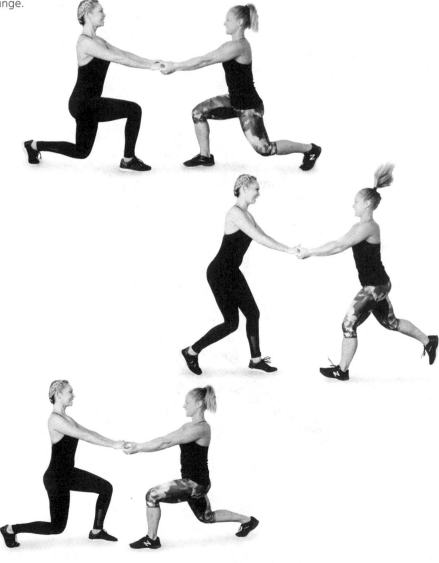

Rotating Plank

1. Start in a High Plank position, side by side.

2. Open your bodies toward each other into a Side Plank with your right arm and your partner's left arm raised. Check out each other's body alignment so that you are in the correct position; this will be when your feet are stacked on top of each other and your feet, hips, and head are in a straight line.

3. Hold for about ten seconds.

4. Return to the High Plank position, then switch to a Side Plank, this time facing away from each other.

5. Hold for about ten seconds.

6. Repeat for the full minute.

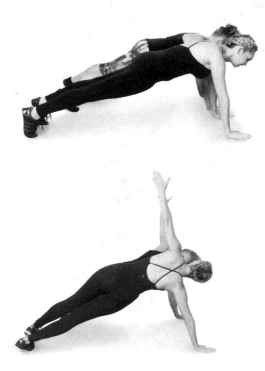

Triceps + Abs Throw Combo

1. Partner A lies on the floor while Partner B straddles their head.

2. Partner A grabs on to Partner B's ankles and extends their legs straight up over their hips.

3. Partner B tries to push Partner A's legs down toward the floor.

4. Partner A resists by engaging their abs while resisting the push, keeping their feet from touching the floor.

5. Repeat the movement and then switch roles after one minute.

TIPS
- Partner A on the floor will be working their abs.
- Partner B will be working their triceps.

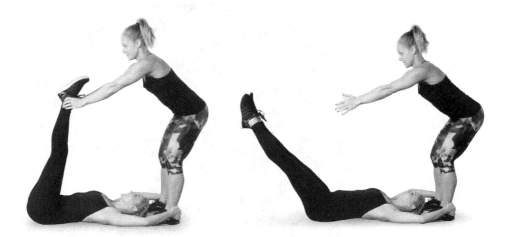

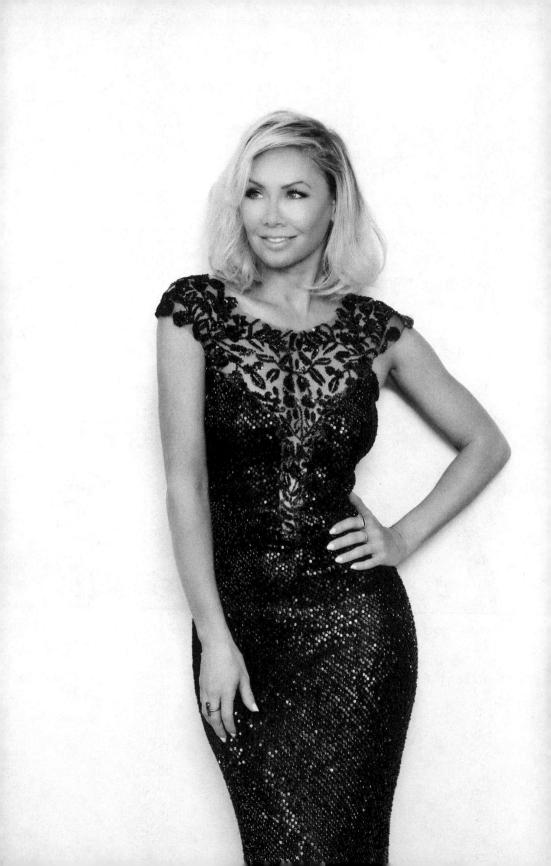

PART IV

The 5-6-7-8 Entertainment Plan

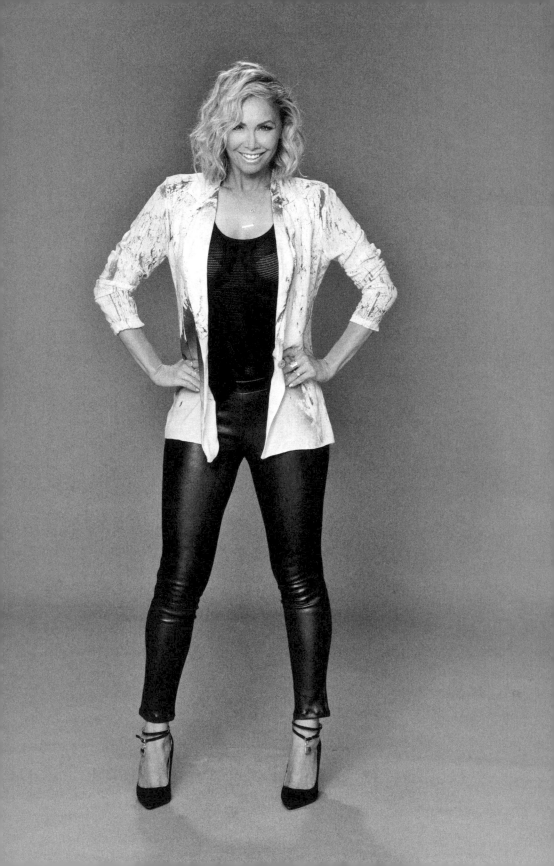

(11)

Fearless Entertaining

Back when I was still a teenager, teaching ballroom dance and doing my training to work at the hotel, one of my college courses was "Food and Beverage." Let's just say this was not my strongest subject. I was much more adept at using the stick shift in the hotel's minivan than I ever was at serving the meals! I still have this vivid memory of taking a tray to a couple who had just checked in after a long flight. We didn't have a trolley, so we had to carry the large trays on our shoulders. I got to the door and tapped it with my foot and said, "Room service." They opened the door and I walked in and was so proud that I got there without spilling anything, but as I entered the room I must have tilted my wrist and the food went flying everywhere. I was so mortified as I knelt down to scoop up the bits of the fish that had been so beautifully grilled and arranged on the plates a minute before. The guests were furious, and I certainly didn't blame them. Honestly, I was the worst waitress ever! So I was put back behind the front desk where I belonged, and from then on everyone got their dinners in one piece.

After the fish ended up on the floor in a big gooey mess, I had a bit of fear about entertaining. It wasn't so much a fear of dropping things, I just didn't have confidence in my cooking or presentation skills. Give me a ballroom dancer's gown and I can decorate it till it's glistening and gorgeous, but give me a plate of veggies to arrange and my mind would go blank!

I think this came about, too, because, like many other dancers I've met, I never spent any time in the kitchen when I was growing up. I was just too busy taking classes after school. Mum made all the healthy meals for the family. I was very lucky that my uncle had a vegetable patch, so we always had fresh vegetables with our meals. Mum would cut up carrot sticks, as I loved to eat them, and I'd take a bag of them to dance class in case I needed a snack. And as Mum cooked, my brother would help her. (And guess what? He's now a professional chef!) So I would get home late from classes and actually eat by myself in front of the TV, as my family had already had their supper. I know, I know—not a great habit, but it didn't bother me. I was so hungry by the time I got home I could have eaten in the garage and been happy!

I wouldn't consider myself a "foodie." I'm very happy with clean, simple meals and just never had the inclination to know how to make anything fancy or complicated. Unfortunately, this didn't translate well to entertaining guests at brunch or dinnertime. It was especially frustrating because I also wanted to share my love of healthy, nutritious meals with my fellow dancers, who ate much of the same foods I did, but I just didn't know how.

When I moved to America and got my apartment in Los Angeles, I decided it was time to finally start cooking. I wanted my friends to hang out and enjoy a meal with me, but I was so nervous about cooking because I wanted to please everybody. I was worried that they wouldn't think it was any good. I didn't even know what plate to put things on for presentation. Of course, I've since learned that the best part of any dinner party is the company, not the food, but that took quite a while to sink in! Entertaining is really about getting the right mix of people more than the right mix of food.

Once, I had a date with someone I really liked, and one of my friends told me I should cook for him. Big mistake. I found a recipe that sounded easy, for chicken in a mushroom white wine sauce with some veggies on the side. I was petrified I would mess up. And so, of course, I messed up. The chicken was undercooked and the veggies were overcooked—or maybe it was the other way around!—and they looked awful. Fortunately, we had a good laugh about it, and I did go on a second date with him—only he suggested that we go out to dinner instead!

Thank goodness a dear friend named Glenn—we grew up together in Sydney—moved to Los Angeles. He's always been a great cook, and he taught me a lot of simple techniques and shortcuts. When we cook together I always learn something new and appreciate how much fun cooking can be. He took away the fear factor because he was there with me, and he didn't care if I messed up. We could always eat the results and no one else would ever know! I just had to do it.

That's when it hit me: Entertaining is just like dancing. You have to have a rehearsal, which is you understanding the fundamentals of cooking and the particular recipes you're going to be making. You start small—with eggs, for example, I got really good at frittatas yet still wouldn't dream of making a soufflé! You get the right equipment. And you give it a shot. If you mess up, you go back to basics and try again.

Then, when it's party time, you become the choreographer and set designer. I want to give my guests the razzle-dazzle in my apartment— even if they're just coming over for a simple, short meal—the same way I'd give it to them onstage. I make sure my place looks pretty. I always get fresh flowers, even if I just pick them from my garden, and arrange the bouquet. I light some scented candles or bake a yummy dessert so it smells divine the minute I open the door to greet my guests. I choose the music and arrange the lighting.

I learned many of those tips from my wonderful friend Carson Kressley, and he's been kind enough to share his best ones on page 268 in this chapter. He's a professional party planner and he is a marvel at it. One day, we went to the gym, and then I invited him over afterward. "Let's make brunch," he said, as he opened my cupboards and refrigerator, peering at what I had in there. "Leave it to me." He sent me to my room and I showered and got ready. Before I knew it, he'd whipped up an omelet, made a salad with a fresh vinaigrette, carved a watermelon into a basket, made a glorious arrangement of flowers from my garden, found my best tablecloth, and lit the candles. I came out of my room to find my apartment transformed. In less than half an hour!

"How did you do that?" I asked him, astonished.

He just smiled. "It's so easy!" he replied.

And once he showed me what to do, it was! Follow these tips, and you'll see how easy entertaining is, too. I put on my apron; everything is set in its place; I've already choreographed the beginning, the middle, and the end in my mind. Time to execute . . . and a five, six, seven, eight!

Be Prepared

One of the reasons why I had so much trouble entertaining is I didn't know how to budget enough time for preparation. It's funny that I even used to think that way, because I was so used to rehearsing over and over again until my dances were perfect. I just never thought to apply that strategy to the kitchen.

This is the best way to prepare:

- Pick your recipes days or even weeks ahead of your party and keep them simple, unless you are an experienced cook.

- Make a shopping list and be sure to take it with you when you go to get the food!

- Test the recipe by cooking it, or choose one you've made before with great success. That way you'll know how long it takes, how it tastes, and whether this is the best dish or not. Do the same kind of tasks (chopping, slicing, arranging) enough times that they become second nature. If you don't like it or it's too complicated and you know it will stress you out, choose something else.

- Make a list of all the things that need to be done.

- Take out all the equipment you need. If your knives, cutting board, pans, and measuring spoons as well as all your food ingredients are in front of you, it's much easier to follow the recipe.

- Do as much as you can the day before. You can clean the house, set the table, put out the wine, and even cook some of the dishes (most food tastes better the next day anyway), especially dessert.

- Clean as you go. That is such an important part of cooking, especially if you have a small kitchen. I really hate to see a pile of dirty dishes in the sink, so I do as much of the washing up or loading of the dishwasher as possible while I'm cooking.

- The day of the party, put on some music that you love as it will always put you in a good mood for cooking and getting ready.

- Do as much as you can in the morning. For example, I often serve cheese platters for those who like savory desserts, and the cheeses taste so much better if they're at room temperature, so I put them out early, with crackers nearby.

- Get yourself ready hours before. I do my hair and makeup and choose my outfit. That way I don't have to worry about dashing off to my room for my lipstick when guests are arriving!

Make One-Pot Meals, Especially in a Slow Cooker

The last thing you want when you're entertaining is to be glued to the stove, stirring a sauce or watching something cook. Once I learned how to use a slow cooker, it made entertaining for a crowd so much easier. I made all the dishes the day before—and basically all I had to do was throw everything into the cooker, put the lid on, turn it to high or low, and leave. I'd come home at the end of the day to an apartment that smelled heavenly, and the bulk of my cooking was done. Even better, if you put the pot in the refrigerator overnight, any fat will rise to the surface and congeal, and it's easy to just skim it off. This makes even high-fat meat dishes so much lower in calories.

If you don't want to use a slow cooker, you can just as easily make one-pot meals. A big pot of spaghetti sauce or a pan full of veggie lasagna or a beef stew are perfect for a crowd. You can make them the day before and reheat them, too.

Have a Go-To Meal

I love having a roast dinner. It's something my family grew up having and it's a very Australian tradition. My mum would make roast lamb with mint sauce and serve it with vegetables. It was so comforting, so delicious, and so healthy—and it was also about our family being together.

As you'll see in the recipes beginning on page 272, my go-to meal is often a roast dinner, because I've made it so many times by now that I never have to worry about it. Roasting the veggies is super easy and it's hard to botch it, unless I forget to take them out of the oven! Everything is so colorful and my table looks lovely when I put the various dishes out. And I find that my guests tend to eat more veggies than meat, which is great for their waistlines.

Potlucks Take the Pressure Off

One trick for easy entertaining is to have a potluck, where you ask your guests to bring a dish. Those who like to cook will whip up one of their go-to dishes, and those who don't can bring drinks or a dessert from a bakery or store. Knowing that other guests will be bringing delicious dishes takes off all the pressure of worrying about your own cooking, and it makes the meal even more fun when there's a wide array of yummy things to eat.

Serve Simple Drinks

I've found that most people like simple drinks when I entertain. Many dancers and performers I know choose not to drink alcohol, so I always have a setup of fizzy waters and juices. I love to put out sliced limes or cucumbers or berries next to the fizzy water, so people can make their own flavored drinks.

For those who do like to drink, I usually serve champagne when they arrive. I'll have vodka out, too, as many of my friends like a vodka and soda since it's very refreshing and low calorie. (You already know not to drink your calories; some mixed cocktails contain over five hundred calories, and I'd much rather eat those calories!) Also, I have a few bottles of red or white wine and some beer on hand. That's it. If you want to stock your bar, go ahead, but most people tend to stick to wine or water at a dinner party.

Set a Beautiful Table Because You Deserve It

Do you have good silverware and dinnerware? If so, do you use them every day? I hope so! I think that the ambiance of your environment when you're eating is often just as important as what's on your plate. You work hard and you deserve to eat in a beautiful setting. It will help you eat more slowly and it will help you sit back and relax, which is not only better for your digestion but very necessary to help you unwind after a stressful day.

Setting a beautiful table is part of mindful eating. It means you are deliberately enticing all of your senses as part of mealtime. So please promise me that you are never going to eat standing up at the kitchen counter. And you are never going to eat on plastic or paper plates unless you are at an outdoor picnic or a child's birthday party!

I make a special point of saying this because I spent so many years on the road, where all too often the only place for me to have a meal was in an anonymous hotel room. Sure, if I ordered room service it would come on a nice trolley with a starched white tablecloth and heavy silver forks (one of the reasons why room service is so nice!), but it wasn't homey. It wasn't my table settings or my water glasses.

My table always looks welcoming, even if I'm eating alone. I light the candles and set out flowers, and I admire how lovely it looks before I start to eat. When I am on my own, my sweet little dog, Lola, will join me—she is the perfect dinner companion! I let her sit at the table on her own special chair because she is very well trained. She gets her own dinner and never begs for mine. (This is a dog who will eat any-thing! She even loves cherry tomatoes and other veggies.) Lola was so shocked when I started cooking, because she couldn't understand why I was spending so much time in the kitchen. Now, of course, her tail starts wagging wildly when I pull out the pots and pans, because she knows it means we're going to have a wonderful dinner together.

Dress for Success in the Kitchen!

I've spent most of my life onstage, wearing an incredible array of costumes. So I like to dress for the part—it truly did help me get into the cooking.

All I did was buy some really cute aprons. One is decorated with cherries and another is covered in cupcakes. I love tying one on and getting to work. I dress for success in the kitchen and I'm instantly in the mood. And my clothes never get grimy, either!

Make It Fun

Because I used to worry so much about cooking, it was never fun for me. Not until Glenn and Carson guided me and taught me what to do did I finally relax in the kitchen. Their enthusiasm was infectious. They were truly enjoying themselves even if we had to peel a huge mountain of potatoes or chop so many onions my eyes were streaming.

Mostly, we had fun because we were doing it together. This is especially important if you're a newbie cook and worried about how high to turn up the burner or when something is cooked through or how to salvage a pot of overcooked pasta. Invite a friend over when you're learning, and go for it together. We tie on our aprons and have a glass of wine, and before we know it the meal is done. And then it's even more fun to eat!

Carson Kressley's Entertainment Tips

You love hosting dinner parties and having friends together. What's the most important piece of advice you'd give to someone who is scared to cook for a large group?

Keep it simple! No one expects you to be a gourmet cook—so keep the food simple. Serving something you know and love takes the fear out of preparing it. I find that people just love an interesting mix of guests and then a simple but delicious menu. For example, at my apartment in New York I'll whip up some comfort food like Bill Blass's meatloaf recipe and some smashed cauliflower and a big salad and serve it on fancy china for a bit of humor. People love it!

What is your go-to menu when you're hosting friends?
It really depends on the season and the occasion. I always try to use foods that are in season. It just feels right and makes sense. Then I keep the spread (giggle) limited to three to five items. A small array of great foods works better together and tastes better than a smorgasbord of random choices. Again, it's about keeping it simple.

What accessories do you use to make the event special?
I always use lovely dinnerware. We are always so rushed and very rarely eat off nice plates anymore! Now, don't get confused. They don't have to be fancy, fine china. They could be mix-and-match from a discount store, flea market finds, or family heirlooms. Just make sure they are nice quality! You deserve it, as do your guests! It's all about making people feel special and taken care of. I always make sure I have a fun table-scape too. This could be fresh flowers or fruits and veggies from my garden. For holidays maybe I'll amp it up and use fun objects to make the table extra special. Disco balls, anyone?

What's your favorite holiday and why?
I just love summer. It's my favorite time of the year. I love being at my horse farm in Pennsylvania during the summer and throwing a big Fourth of July barbecue. I'll grill good old hot dogs (all-beef from a local Amish butcher) and great-quality sirloin burgers. Then I'll whip up a few classics like German potato salad (no mayo!) and deviled eggs to round things out. Guests just relax in the pool while I grill, and then we graze and have local sparkling Pinot sangria!

What advice did you first give Kym when she moved into her own place and started cooking?
Get the right tools: good knives and a good set of pots and pans. Then just start slow and simple and have fun with it! It worked.

What makes an outstanding host or hostess?
Making everyone feel like the guest of honor. Make sure they have a drink right away and keep checking in to make sure they always feel well

taken care of. I keep my parties on the smaller side so that I can check in with everyone!

What are your "must haves" for a great event?
A great playlist—sometimes I'm lazy and just use Pandora. I'm wild about Captain and Tennille radio! Simple but delicious food and plenty of it. And a fun and diverse group of friends. That's all!

Do you use checklists to organize yourself for an event?
I'm a total list maker. If I'm throwing a party, big or small, you can bet I have a long list of things to do. Here's an example:

- Clean house.
- Prepare as much food as possible the night before.
- Set table.
- Have playlist at the ready.
- Stock the bar.
- Hire a bartender (this sounds extravagant but is so good for bigger parties; they make sure guests are served and you can mingle).
- Decorations
- Candles

How has Kym improved as a hostess over the time you've known her?
Well, I think her first endeavor at hostessing landed her in the emergency room—I wish I was kidding but I'm not! She managed to drop a glass vase as she was drying the dishes and as it broke the glass cut her leg open. She needed so many stitches it was ridiculous. She has the scar to prove it. But now she is relaxed and gracious and quick to have a laugh at her own parties. Those are all hallmarks of a successful host.

Do you like to give away party favors after a dinner party?
I often don't because it's just not necessary, but it is a delightful surprise if you do! How about:

- The evening's playlist on a jump drive
- A mini silver frame that was used as a place card holder
- Homemade cookies for the ride home!

5-6-7-8 Let's Have a Party!

These are several of my favorite occasions for entertaining. I hope your parties will be as much fun as mine!

Kym and Katrina's Barbecue

Australians spend much of their lives outdoors (wearing sunscreen and hats, of course), and our barbecues are a big deal for us. You know the old cliché: "Throw a shrimp on the barbie!" That's our slang at work!

Barbecues are a wonderful way to entertain if you have the space for a good grill. In fact, one of the best birthday gifts I ever got was a big fancy barbecue for my apartment in Los Angeles. My friends, who know I used to be cooking-challenged, were always shocked when they came over for a barbecue, because I'd be fearlessly wielding the tongs. Grilling is so easy, and cooking food over hot coals or gas means a lot of the fat drips away. It's almost impossible to do things wrong unless you misjudge the timing and don't cook your meat for long enough. And it smells so good whenever you light up.

My friend Katrina Brown and I often have barbecues at my house in Los Angeles. She's a boxer and when she's training full-time to prepare her body for fighting she knows how important it is to eat clean and fresh food. "I focus most of my meals around protein and greens," she told me, "and I follow two main elements: The first is to eat organic from the local farmer's market. When I do, my body functions so much more fluidly on all levels—my skin is clean and glowing, my moods are more stable, and my energy levels are consistent. The other element that I like to follow is barbecuing my produce, which I love."

Follow these recipes and you can have a healthy barbecue with extra-delicious veggies. The high heat helps caramelize the natural sugars in them so they become super sweet.

Grilled Meat

Serves: At least 4, with leftovers

Ingredients

1–2 pounds meat of your choice (It's better to cook a lot since the grill is hot and add the leftovers to salads or snacks the next day.)

4 tablespoons organic barbecue sauce per piece of meat

1 teaspoon paprika

Salt and pepper

1. Put the meat in a glass bowl or container and add barbecue sauce. Add paprika and salt and pepper to taste.
2. Cover tightly and marinate for several hours or overnight.
3. Grill meat until thoroughly cooked. The timing will depend on the thickness of the meat—usually no more than 10–15 minutes. Turn the pieces often. Chicken should be cooked until the juices run clear. Discard marinade (it has raw meat juices in it).

Salad

You can use whichever mix of greens you like.

Serves: 4

Ingredients

1 bunch kale

1 bunch spinach

1 head butter lettuce

$1/4$ cup dried cranberries

$1/4$ cup crumbled goat cheese, feta cheese, blue cheese, or other cheese of your choice

$1/4$–$1/2$ cup thinly sliced almonds

Vinaigrette (recipe on page 118)

1. Wash the kale, spinach, and butter lettuce thoroughly. Dry and shred into small pieces. Place in a large serving bowl.
2. Add dried cranberries, cheese, and almonds. Toss gently.
3. Add vinaigrette or serve it on the side.

Grilled Veggies

For quantities: Use however much you like, depending on how many guests you have.

Serves: At least 4

Ingredients

1–2 eggplants	2–3 sweet potatoes or yams
2–3 red peppers	Coconut oil, liquid or spray
2–3 onions	Cinnamon (optional)
2–3 zucchini	Chili flakes (optional)

1. Slice eggplants into thin slices. You don't need to peel them.
2. Slice red peppers and remove all seeds.
3. Slice onions.
4. Cut zucchini into long strips.
5. Peel and slice sweet potatoes or yams into thick cubes or rounds.
6. Boil a pot full of water and drop in all the veggies. Cook for 5–8 minutes, until softened. (This step will shorten the cooking time, but it isn't mandatory.) Drain well and rub in about $1/2$ teaspoon of coconut oil. Sprinkle with just a touch of cinnamon if you want them sweet, or a few chili flakes if you want them spicy.
7. When the grill is hot, spray on a fine mist of coconut oil to prevent the veggies from sticking. Or you can also use a pastry brush and apply a sheer coating to the veggies, too.
8. Grill until tender, turning often. This should take no more than 15 minutes. (If you didn't parboil the veggies, they will take longer.)

Roast Dinner for Four

As you read earlier in this chapter, one of my favorite childhood memories is our family roast dinners. It wasn't what we ate that was so important, even though my mother's cooking was terrific, but that we were all together, sitting round our dining room table and talking and eating and enjoying each other's company.

A roast dinner is very easy to make. Basically, you turn on the oven, put in the meat and veggies, and then wait for them to be cooked! We often ate roast lamb but I find that a roast chicken is one of my go-to meals. You can experiment with using different seasonings on the skin, or adding a lemon or orange to the cavity for extra flavor. It's also very easy to double or triple the quantities if you're having a lot of people over.

Roast Chicken

One of the easiest and most satisfying roasts to make! Any leftover meat can be shredded and used in salads the next day, and you can even simmer the bones with some cut-up veggies for a few hours to make chicken stock, if you're feeling adventurous.

Serves: 4

Ingredients

1 2–3 pound roasting chicken
$1/2$ tablespoon olive oil
1 lime, halved
Salt and pepper
4 garlic cloves
1 branch of rosemary

1. Preheat oven to 375 degrees.
2. Rinse off chicken and dry thoroughly. Rub olive oil into skin. Squeeze on the juice of half the lime and rub it in. Season with salt and pepper.
3. Place garlic cloves, rosemary, and the remaining lime half in the cavity of the chicken.
4. Roast for 35–45 minutes, depending on the size of the chicken. (It's cooked when the leg moves easily and the juices run clear when you prick the chicken with a fork.)

Roast Pork or Turkey Fillets

Another super-easy roast to make is a pork loin or turkey breast. I was thrilled to see these in supermarkets when I moved to Los Angeles, as they were already packaged and ready to go. Loins of pork and turkey are high in protein and low in fat, and these roasts are inexpensive and will give you lots of meat for leftovers, too.

Serves: 4

Ingredients

2 pork or turkey fillets

2 tablespoons olive oil, divided

6 white potatoes, cubed (no need to peel)

1 large sweet potato, peeled and roughly chopped

2 carrots, chopped

1 small butternut squash, peeled and cubed

3 small zucchini, sliced

Salt and pepper

1. Preheat oven to 400 degrees.
2. Sear pork or turkey in a frying pan with 1 tablespoon of olive oil.*
3. Transfer pork or turkey to a cookie sheet with a high rim or to a baking pan with a wire rack so the meat sits on that. Roast for 45 minutes.
4. Remove the pan from the oven. Toss cut-up vegetables with remaining 1 tablespoon olive oil. Add to pan.
5. Return the pan to the oven. Bake 1 hour, stirring the vegetables well at least once.
6. Season with salt and pepper to taste.

---

* If you're in a super hurry you can omit this step, but it does make the meat taste better!

Roast Fish

This is extremely simple and delicious. I think fish tastes better when it's roasted rather than sautéed, and it cooks very quickly. Experiment with different seasonings; the rosemary pairs well with the lemon, but if you prefer paprika or curry, for example, sprinkle on a bit and omit the lemon. This is one of the few occasions where I like to use butter rather than olive oil, but you can swap if you like.

Serves: 4

Ingredients

Cooking spray

2 pounds boned fish fillet of your choice (cod, red snapper, salmon, etc.)

2 tablespoons butter, cut into small pieces

2 sprigs rosemary (optional)

Salt and pepper, to taste

1. Preheat oven to 400 degrees.
2. Spray baking pan with cooking spray to oil it.
3. Place half the lemon slices in the pan and lay the fish, skin-side down, atop them.
4. Dot the fish with butter. Place rosemary and remaining lemon slices on top.
5. Bake for about 20 minutes, or until the fish is opaque.

Roast Vegetables

Roasting veggies caramelizes their natural sugars and makes them even more delicious. You can use any mixture of veggies that you like. Chop them roughly to save time—they don't have to look perfect. Be sure to stir them often so they don't stick to the pan!

Serves: 4

Ingredients

2 zucchini, chopped	2 sweet potatoes, peeled and chopped
2 carrots, chopped	1 large red onion, chopped
$1/2$ pound Brussels sprouts, trimmed and halved	8 cloves garlic, peeled and halved
	2 tablespoons coconut oil
$1/2$ pound butternut squash, peeled and chopped	2 sprigs fresh rosemary or thyme
	Sea salt

1. Preheat oven to 400 degrees.
2. Place veggies on a roasting tray, drizzle with oil (coconut oil must be in liquid form; if yours has solidified, which coconut oil can do if the kitchen isn't particularly warm, heat it for about 20–30 seconds in the microwave, or until it melts), and season with herbs and salt.
3. Roast in the oven until tender, about 30 minutes.

Cauliflower Cheese

The first time I mentioned to my American friends that I was having Cauliflower Cheese for lunch, they looked a bit bewildered. "How can cheese be made out of cauliflower?" one of them finally asked as I laughed. "Sorry!" I replied. "In Australia, when we say this, we mean a veggie cooked with a cheese sauce." This is one of my mum's specialties, and I've tweaked it to cut down on the fat content. It's just as yummy this way!

Serves: 4

Ingredients

Cooking spray
1 medium head cauliflower, cut into florets
1 tablespoon butter
I pinch salt
1 tablespoon flour
1 cup skim milk
1 teaspoon Dijon or spicy mustard
$^{1}/_{2}$ cup sharp reduced-fat cheese (can be cheddar or Swiss), shredded or cut into small pieces

1. Preheat oven to 400 degrees. Spray a baking dish with cooking spray.
2. In a saucepan, steam cauliflower florets for 4–5 minutes. (You can also do this in the microwave with $^{1}/_{2}$ cup water for 3–4 minutes.) Drain and place cauliflower florets into baking dish.
3. Melt butter with a pinch of salt in a small saucepan over low heat. Add the flour and stir until smooth and there are no lumps.
4. Add the milk. Continue to stir until the sauce thickens. Stir in the mustard.
5. Pour the sauce over the cauliflower and sprinkle the cheese on top.
6. Bake for 15 minutes.

Italian Dinner

An Italian dinner is something to consider when you don't want to spend a lot of time in the kitchen. The meatballs and ratatouille can be made the day before and will taste even better the next day. One of the easiest dishes to make for a dinner party is this one, given to me by Carson Kressley. Of course you can make regular spaghetti for friends who aren't on the 5-6-7-8 Diet Plan, but I think it tastes so much better with spaghetti squash.

Katrina's Zucchini Spaghetti

My friend Katrina taught me this recipe. It's very flavorful. She likes to add some fresh peas on top if they're in season, to make it even greener.

Serves: 4

Ingredients

4 zucchini

4 ounces fresh pesto sauce

1. If you have a food processor, thinly slice or shred zucchini. Otherwise, cut into very fine strips.
2. Lightly steam zucchini for 3–4 minutes in a saucepan until al dente. You can also use a microwave and $1/4$ cup water for 2–3 minutes.
3. Drain zucchini and top with pesto sauce. Mix gently and serve immediately.

Carson's Spaghetti Squash and Meatballs

To serve, add a jar of high-quality marinara sauce and 6 basil leaves, chopped.

Serves: 4

Ingredients for Meatballs

1¹/₂ pounds ground turkey

1 teaspoon salt

¹/₂ teaspoon pepper

1 egg, beaten

1 small onion, diced

¹/₂ cup fresh Italian parsley, chopped

¹/₂ cup Italian bread crumbs

1 tablespoon olive oil

1. Mix all the ingredients except for the olive oil well. You can use your hands if you like!
2. Form the mixture into small balls.
3. Heat olive oil over medium heat and sauté meatballs for about 10–15 minutes, until thoroughly cooked.

Ingredients for Spaghetti Squash

1 medium spaghetti squash

1 tablespoon olive oil

Salt and pepper

1. Pierce five or six holes in the top of the squash as vents. Microwave for about 8 minutes. Adjust microwaving time if the squash is extra large or small.
2. Carefully remove the squash from the microwave and slice lengthwise. Be careful as it's been steaming inside!
3. Remove the seeds and scoop the flesh out—as you do it will form spaghetti-like strands. Dress with olive oil, and salt and pepper to taste.

Florence Henderson's Lemon Pasta with Almonds

This is simple and elegant.

Serves: 4

Ingredients

1 pound fresh pasta

1 tablespoon olive oil

Grated zest of 1 lemon

1 tablespoon fresh lemon juice

$^1/_2$ cup chopped almonds

$^1/_4$ cup crumbled feta cheese

1. Cook pasta in boiling water until al dente.

2. Toss with remaining ingredients, except for feta cheese.

3. Add feta cheese and toss gently. Serve hot.

Florence Henderson's Ratatouille

This isn't Italian, but it's a wonderful dish for a party. Many French recipes for ratatouille contain copious amounts of oil—but Florence is an experienced cook who has removed most of it with no loss of flavor. When you're buying eggplants, the smaller the better, as the larger ones can get bitter. And you don't have to peel small ones either.

Serves: 4

Ingredients

2 tablespoons olive oil

3–4 cloves garlic, crushed (just smash them with the bottom of a heavy can or bottle and the peel comes right off!)

2 medium yellow onions, chopped

2 small or 1 medium eggplant, cut into 1-inch chunks

4 zucchini, cut into $1/2$- to 1-inch chunks

1 green pepper, cored, seeded, and cut into $1/2$-inch chunks

1 14.5-ounce can of Italian-style tomatoes, chopped

2 tablespoons balsamic vinegar

$1/4$ cup pitted black olives, halved

2 teaspoons dried Italian herb seasoning

Salt and pepper

$1/2$ cup Parmesan, freshly grated

1. Heat olive oil in a large saucepan over medium heat. Add garlic and onion and cook, stirring often, until translucent, about 4–5 minutes.
2. Add eggplant and cook, stirring often, for 2–3 minutes.
3. Stir in the zucchini, green pepper, and tomatoes, and cook, stirring, for 5 minutes more.
4. Add the balsamic vinegar, olives, Italian herb seasoning, and salt and pepper to taste. Reduce the heat to medium-low and stir well.
5. Cover and cook until the vegetables are softened, about 5 minutes more.
6. Remove from heat and pour into a serving bowl. Top with Parmesan cheese. Serve hot.

Teatime Tea Party

You already know how much I love my teas—any time is teatime, especially the 5-6-7-8 way! High tea is usually served at four in the afternoon, and the traditional one is a full meal. You'll be given plates of scones with thick clotted cream, savories like mini quiches and cucumber sandwiches (on white bread, with the crust cut off, if you please!), pots of hot tea with milk and sugar, and lots of little desserts. It's an English and Australian experience, to be sure, but one that can wreak havoc on your calorie intake and digestion!

So why not have your own tea party with my therapeutic teas? Serve any of the delicious savory snacks from the recipes in chapter 5, and any of these desserts. You will be just as satisfied, believe me!

SUGGESTED SAVORIES

- See pages 123 to 125 in chapter 5 for snack ideas.

- Hollow out an avocado and fill with tuna salad.

- Top rice crackers with natural peanut butter.

- Make lettuce wraps with tuna salad, egg salad, chicken breast, or turkey breast inside.

- Cut up organic tofu into small squares and toss with a teaspoon of curry powder and two-thirds of a cup Greek yogurt.

- Strawberries or raspberries in nonfat cottage cheese.

SUGGESTED SWEETS

Australian Pavlova

A Pavlova is one of the best-known of all the Australian desserts—what we call puddings. The original version was created for the ballerina Anna Pavlova during one of her tours in Australia and New Zealand in the 1920s and is typically served with loads of whipped cream on top. I've cut the cream way down, and, actually, you don't need it at all as the meringue and the fruit are luscious and sweet—and fat-free!

Serves: 4

Ingredients

4 egg whites

Salt, a few pinches

1 cup superfine or caster sugar (if you can't find these sugars in the grocery store, pulverize regular granulated sugar in a food processor or blender for 2 minutes until it's very, very fine—this step really is essential!)

1 teaspoon white vinegar

1 teaspoon pure vanilla

1 tablespoon flour

6 teaspoons fresh cream

2 passion fruits, papayas, or mangoes, diced

2 cups mixed berries

1. Preheat oven to 400 degrees. Line two large baking trays or cookie sheets with parchment baking paper.
2. With an electric mixer, beat egg whites with a few pinches of salt for 5–6 minutes, gradually adding the sugar until the mixture becomes thick and glossy. Gently stir in the vinegar and vanilla.
3. Sift the flour over the mixture. Using a large metal spoon, gently fold the flour in.
4. Use the metal spoon to heap dollops of the mixture onto the parchment-lined trays. Try to keep each spoonful circular in shape, and create a shallow dip in the center of each.
5. Turn the oven down to 250 degrees and place the Pavlovas in the oven. Bake for 30 minutes.
6. Once the Pavlovas are cooked, turn the oven off and leave them in the oven until they have cooled completely.
7. When ready to serve, whip the cream. Place a small spoonful of the cream in the center of each Pavlova. Then swirl the passion fruit, papaya, or mango on top of cream. Top each with a small mixture of berries.

Note: I know what you're thinking—cream? You can absolutely forgo the cream and simply place the fruit on top of the Pavlovas. I'll admit, though, that it's not really a proper Australian Pavlova without the cream, and even I give in sometimes and add it!

Apple Raspberry Crumble

This dessert is extremely delicious and is heavy on the fruit and very light on the topping. You can try making it with other combinations of fruit and berries, such as peaches and blueberries or nectarines and pitted cherries, too.

Serves: 4

Ingredients

4 apples

4 tablespoons butter, softened, divided

2 teaspoons plus 2 tablespoons brown sugar

1 teaspoon cinnamon

2 containers raspberries

4 tablespoons whole-wheat flour

2 tablespoons unsweetened shredded coconut

Cooking spray

1. Preheat oven to 325 degrees.
2. Peel, slice, and quarter the apples.
3. Melt 2 of the tablespoons of butter in a pan and sauté apples over medium heat. Add 2 teaspoons brown sugar and the cinnamon, and stir. Pour in the raspberries and gently stir.
4. In a bowl stir together the flour, shredded coconut, and 2 tablespoons of brown sugar. Add the remaining 2 tablespoons of butter.
5. Use your fingers or two forks to crumble the mixture together until well blended.
6. Spray cooking spray into an 8-inch pie tin. Place the fruit mixture into the pie tin, then top with the crumble. Place the tin on a cookie sheet and bake for about 15 minutes until the top starts to brown.
7. Serve warm.

Fruity Applesauce

This is so easy to make and it's best when you make a large batch—I get apples at the local farmers' market, where they sell bags of the less-than-perfect ones for a very low price. Freeze whatever you aren't serving. It's especially filling when eaten while warm and is a terrific substitute when you're craving something soft and sweet, like ice cream—there's no added sugar. If you're using the orange juice, you omit the lemon and use an orange instead.

Serves: At least 4–6

Ingredients

1 5-pound bag apples

1 lemon, halved

1 bag fresh cranberries

1 cup raisins

1 cup apple cider, orange juice, or water

1. Core the apples and cut into chunks. You don't need to peel them. Place them in a large pot.
2. Squeeze the lemons over the apples to get out most of the juice and add the lemon halves to the pot.
3. Add the fresh cranberries, raisins, and liquid to the pot and stir well.
4. Cook over medium heat until the liquid starts to boil. Stir well, and turn heat to medium-low.
5. Cook until the apples are very soft, about 45 minutes to 1 hour. Stir often to make sure nothing's sticking to the bottom of the pot. The apples will reduce as they cook.
6. When cooked, you can make the applesauce smoother by pureeing in a blender or food processor, but I think it's better when it's chunky. Serve warm or cold.

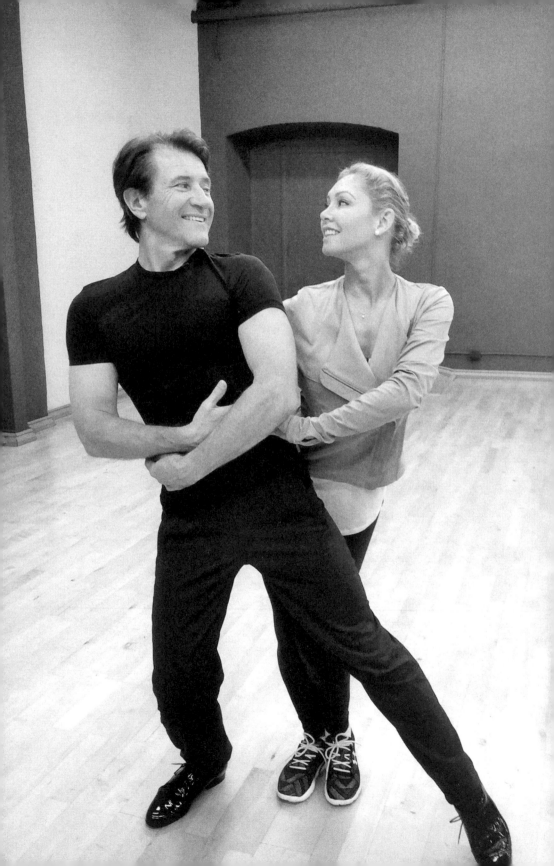

PART V

Unexpected Romance

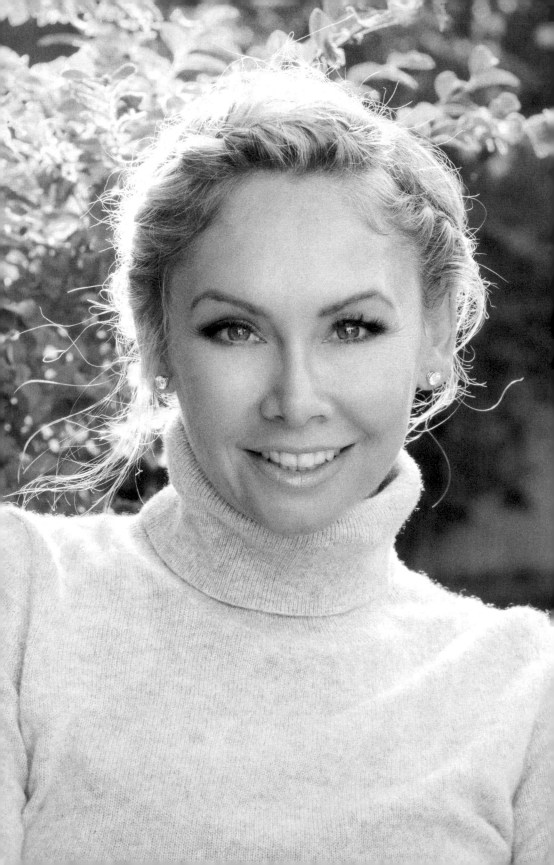

12

Trust the Timing of Your Life

I have always been an old-fashioned romantic girl. Maybe it was growing up watching all those classic MGM musicals that instilled my love for dreaming about the one. Still, I have had some not-so-great relationships in my life. In one instance, I stayed in a bad relationship for much longer than I should have because I tried to convince myself that I'd made the choice of my own free will, so I should stick it out. I wanted it to work so I could almost prove myself right that it was the best option for me. I had always been very strong. I knew who I was and what I wanted. I was taught to have a strong sense of self-worth, as you know.

But something was different in this relationship. I guess you could say this was a time in my life when I lost my way. When that happens and you end a tough relationship, it's important to turn to your friends and family. They love you through thick and thin, and I honestly don't know how I could have moved on without their guidance and support.

Another time, I was engaged and made the very difficult

decision to end this relationship, just before leaving Australia to join the American version of *Dancing with the Stars*. He was a lovely man but I just was not ready for marriage. I lived with a lot of regret for a while and hated myself for hurting someone so much. It all worked out for the best, though.

When I was working on *Dancing with the Stars* in Los Angeles, I was really happy pursuing my dreams but very lonely at times, too. I then met a lovely man and had a great relationship with him. We were friends first, then started dating. I was in my early thirties and thinking about marriage and kids. I thought he was too, but when I asked questions about our future plans he freaked out and broke up with me. It was a hard time as I was no spring chicken anymore. I didn't want to go out and date or do anything. I was worried I would just try to find someone to settle with because time wasn't on my side.

My friends eventually took action and came over to my house one night and told me to get off the couch and come out with them, as I hadn't dated for about a year at that point. I reluctantly did and they jokingly said, "You can't say no. If someone asks you out, no matter what, you have to say yes." Really bad idea! I could see this man approaching me at the bar and I tried to avoid all eye contact. Too late! He was a Hollywood producer, and he asked if he could take me out to dinner and I had to say yes. I was so angry with my friends, but I still went on the date, and all he wanted to talk about was the things he had happening, but nothing had ever happened! He dropped me off at home and that was the last I saw of him, thankfully, as I couldn't wait to be back on my couch with my sweet dog, Lola, and my PJs on.

I also tried a man fast—for three months you can't date, flirt, or think about a man. This seemed to have the opposite effect, though. I would be out shopping or running errands and someone would ask me out. I would say, "I'm sorry, I'm on a man fast and can't"—and it would make them chase me even more!

Let's just say I really was getting fed up with being single in Los Angeles, and I have to admit that I was getting worried I would become bitter and jaded . . . and I certainly did not want to be that kind of person. I've always had a lot of love to give and decided to give it to myself . . . So I made a wholly self-involved decision and froze my eggs. I was nervous about the procedure and about telling my mum this, but she was really supportive.

Off I went to the endocrinologist with my best friend, Glenn, to get more information. I decided to go ahead and I started the process, even though it meant I had to do three injections a day for days. Luckily, Glenn did them for me as I'm a fainter when it comes to needles. After all that, I went for my last ultrasound before the eggs were meant to be harvested, and my doctor told me I hadn't produced enough! I was devastated and told him to try to retrieve whatever he could. Eventually, I chose to undergo the process again, because I knew that while the timing wasn't right for me to have children then, it was most definitely something I wanted down the road. Freezing your eggs isn't for everyone—it is expensive and difficult and painful and may not be something you believe in—but for me it was the right decision. It took the pressure off me with dating and the need to settle. I just know in my heart I want to be a mum one day. That being said, I know there are lots of other ways to be a mum and still don't rule those options out.

Even though I was single and hadn't met the right man and was frustrated and worried, it is not paradoxical to say that I was still happy. It really annoys me when people are so judgmental, especially when they see a single woman in her thirties. "Oh, you poor thing," they say, as if being married is the only goal in life. Certainly, there were times when I was sad or lonely and wanted to be with someone, but I was mostly happy. I had a great job and friends and a home. A lot of my friends are single and very happy, too—and proud to say so.

You need to trust the timing of your life. I would rather be by myself than in a relationship that's awful and making everyone unhappy. Relationships are meant to build on the happiness and love you already have. I'm so glad I never settled and that I stayed true to my heart. Even in my loneliest moments I never gave up on the idea of sharing my life with someone I love and respect and who and loves and respects me back.

So there I was, with my wonderful family and friends, enjoying working on the next phase of my life—big changes that meant hanging up my dance shoes and focusing on health and fitness, and my new role as a *Dancing with the Stars* judge. I was doing a lot of things that made me happy and surrounding myself with people I love. I think that is when you are open to meeting someone. But I was never expecting Robert Herjavec to walk in the door and for me to feel the way I did.

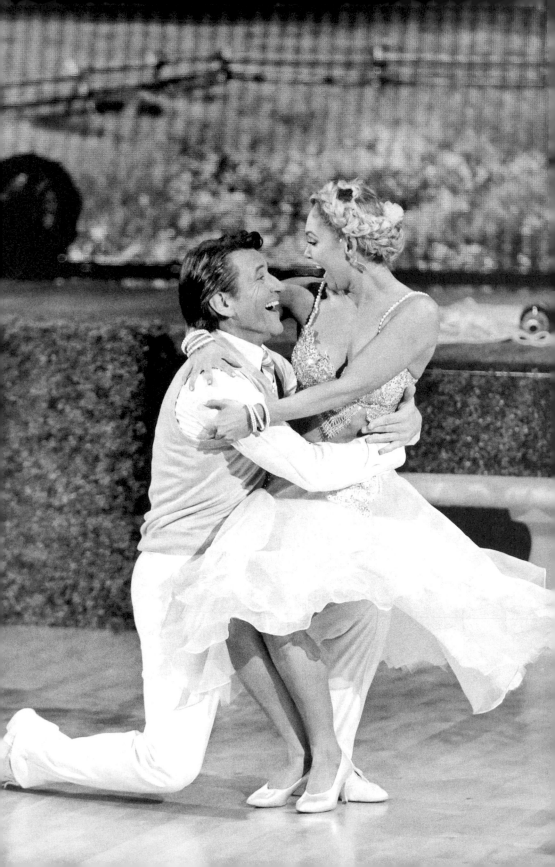

13

Fairy Tales
Do Come True

Out of the blue, in the spring of 2015, I got a phone call from Deena Katz, the executive producer of the American *Dancing with the Stars*. I hadn't been on for a few seasons and was focused on judging in Australia. I'd joined the tour in the US and thought that would be it, so this call was a total surprise.

"We have the perfect partner for you," she told me. "So you have to come back!"

I had no idea at the time that Robert Herjavec had gone to Deena's home for dinner the night before. Robert had been asked to do the show a few months earlier and had agreed but was concerned that Deena didn't know that he was separated from his wife. His kids are so important to him and he often talks about them on *Shark Tank*. The story of his separation had come out, but it hadn't gotten a lot of media attention. While he was thrilled to have been selected to appear on the show, he was so distraught about the end of his marriage that he was considering backing out—because he didn't want the news of the divorce to come out in a bigger way and negatively affect his family, or to create a distraction for the show. Deena reassured him that this would be a positive experience and something that would help him get his energy and spirits back. As he left that night, she turned to her husband and said, "We have to get Kym back on the show. They would be perfect for each other." She just had a feeling. When she told me this, months later, it left me in tears. How lovely that Deena was willing to put us together. I often think back to that moment and wonder where we would both be now if she hadn't made that connection.

The morning I woke up to meet my new dance partner I was more excited than I had ever been. Perhaps it was because I had been off the show for three seasons, or maybe deep down I knew something greater than winning a Mirror Ball was about to happen. As cheesy as it sounds, I just had the feeling that this season was going to be great for me in some regard.

I got to the studio and saw a really fancy car parked around the back, and the staff told me to park in the front as they were filming something with my new partner in the studio (I was hoping to get a sneak peek). I called my friend Carson and told him I didn't yet know who my partner was but that he had a really nice car. Carson asked which type but I had no idea! I was thinking Robert Kennedy Jr. was going to be my partner, but that amazing car had me thinking that perhaps he might be a race car driver! I walked up into the studio to find the producers and crew ready for me. I was fishing for clues but they wouldn't budge! I had no idea who was about to walk through that door. Unfortunately, when he walked in, I still didn't! Well, I am kidding a bit, as I knew he was from *Shark Tank*, but I didn't know his name . . . which was so embarrassing! I do know that the first thing I thought was how handsome and friendly he looked.

Robert and I didn't start dancing straightaway; we had to shoot an introductory segment first. We were told to get into his car, with Robert at the wheel, driving around Los Angeles, so we could have a nice little chat and get to know a bit about each other and break the ice. I had an earpiece in one ear that enabled me to communicate with the producers so they could give me some additional questions to ask and tell me what to elaborate on if they were looking for different topics—this is what happens behind the scenes of a TV show! I was asking the general questions, such as, "Why did you decide to do this?" "Have you ever danced?"—and then he started asking 101 questions about *me*. Where I come from and how I learned to dance and so forth. It really was that moment that the connection happened. I could feel a spark and was hoping he did, too. Then I was snapped back into reality when I heard the producers' voices crackling in my ear, telling me to ask this and that! I talked myself out of those romantic thoughts and went about my job.

After our drive, we went right back to the dance studio because Robert wanted to get started rehearsing straightaway. It was adorable seeing how excited and eager he was to get going—some of my partners had been so nervous that they were more reluctant to start moving. As ever, I didn't know what dance we would have first, so I was just showing him some basic dance moves in order to gauge his level of expertise and see what I was dealing with. I could tell immediately Robert hadn't had any dance experience, but he had something so special that you cannot teach, and that was his personality, enthusiasm, and charm.

I have learned never to mix business with pleasure, so I must confess I was a little freaked out at first. We were both very polite and professional but I could feel there was an attraction there. It was subtle and oh so sweet. It was in the way he looked at me, not just as a professional dancer who was his teacher, but as a woman he found interesting. In the way he tried not to hold my fingers longer than he needed to when I was showing him a turn. In the way that he was always smiling and cheerful and attentive. There was a kind of joy radiating out of him, something that I think surprised him, too. We both felt it before we could put it into words. And I think because we were both so surprised—neither of us went into this particular season expecting anything truly out of the ordinary—by how seamlessly we were meshing that we almost didn't want to do anything to change the energy.

Robert did ask me out to dinner about two weeks into rehearsal. At the time I said yes, but the more I thought about it, the more scared I became. So at the end of rehearsals I casually said, "Oh, about dinner, I'm so sorry but I can't make it tonight. See you for rehearsals tomorrow!" While he was meant to be focusing on the cha-cha that day, I could tell he had been thinking about where he would take me and was excited about this dinner. He went home confused and upset. I did cave in a week later and convinced myself that one meal wasn't going to do any harm. We have to eat, right?

A day or so after I said yes, Robert asked if I would mind if the dinner date actually took place at a wedding. Yes . . . a wedding! I think I was so taken aback and so surprised to have been asked this—after all, going to a wedding is usually a sign of a commitment, and at this point we still barely knew each other—that Robert laughed and quickly explained that it wasn't actually a wedding but a commitment ceremony. Two of his very dear friends had already been married for twenty years and were having a small ceremony to renew their vows. And he wanted me to go with him. Could this possibly have been any more romantic? I don't think so!

I looked at his eager, hopeful smile, and my heart melted. He was just so honest and real and didn't seem like the other men I'd met and dated. Most of them had played games or seemed to have ulterior motives. None of them would ever have asked me to go to a commitment ceremony with them. So I smiled back with what I knew was the same eager hopefulness and told Robert I would be thrilled to go with him.

I will never forget the day Robert came to pick me up. We had been rehearsing all morning and I only had forty-five minutes to dash home and get ready. Which was no time at all, especially considering that I was in a total freak-out about what to wear, and I was a sweaty, hot mess! Thank goodness for my need-to-quick-change dancer training, where I was used to going from one costume to the next in mere minutes before appearing back onstage. I somehow managed to shower, twist up my hair in a dancer's bun as I'd done thousands of times before, dab on a tiny bit of makeup, and pull on one of my faithful little black dresses. To this day Robert still tells people he's amazed at how quickly I can get ready for a formal event. It must be all those thousands of dancer's buns coming in handy, but whenever he says this I have to laugh, because believe me, I was sweating it before that wedding!

I had just finished putting my essentials in my clutch bag when the doorbell rang. I'm not going to lie—by this time the butterflies in my tummy were fluttering like mad and my heart was racing as if I'd just done an entire performance of *Burn the Floor*. I quickly wiped my palms so they wouldn't be too sweaty and opened the door. Robert was standing there looking like an ad for menswear in *GQ*. He was wearing a gorgeous black tuxedo that, as I gushed over it, he told me had been made by Tom Ford. He handed me an enormous bouquet of deep red roses that smelled as intoxicated as I was feeling. It was quite surreal, and I kept having to tell myself to not get swept away!

I invited Robert in for a quick moment so I could put the roses in a vase, and when we walked outside I saw his car. A gleaming black Rolls-Royce was parked outside my house. I can only imagine what my neighbors must have thought! I'd never been in such a luxurious car before.

The drive to the venue took nearly an hour, so we had a lot of time to talk about things. I could tell why Robert is so successful. He asked a lot of unusual questions—not just to make idle chitchat but because he was genuinely interested—and before I knew it, I was telling him many of the details of my life story. He had the most amazing way of making me feel comfortable and relaxed, and that's because he's so genuine and really did want to know all about what made me tick.

Needless to say, the drive was one of the most enjoyable I've ever had. I had no trouble talking to him and he told me some of his story, which I found fascinating, as does everyone who hears it. To escape the repressive Communist regime, Robert had come over on a boat from what was then Yugoslavia (now Croatia) to Canada with his family when he was eight. He spoke no English and his family was so impoverished they lived in the basement apartment of the home of family friends for eighteen months. As he got older, Robert worked at a succession of minimum-wage jobs to put himself through college and help support his family. And after he convinced the head of a start-up technology company to let him work for free, he found his niche and became an incredibly successful entrepreneur in the tech field. But even as his business soared, he never forgot where he came from and the importance of a strong and determined work ethic.

We finally arrived at his friend's house, where the groom met us at the door. We talked for a minute or so and then Robert said a quick good-bye as he had to hurry off to go pick up the bride. I could tell he had misjudged the timing a bit, but told him I was fine and went in and made some new friends. Robert didn't come back for a good hour and half, arriving at my side just as the bride walked down the aisle.

The ceremony itself was so romantic and surreal. Robert was sitting next to me as we watched two beautiful people talk about how they loved each other more on that day than they had when they'd gotten married two decades before. They spoke about how their love never wavered through all the ups and downs that life had thrown at them. It was in that moment that Robert gently put his hand on mine. I nearly died but it felt so right!

What a magical night that was, surrounded by love and friendship and people who truly cared about each other and wanted to share their love with those closest to them. I got to meet some of Robert's dearest friends and see how normal and kind he was. Even though some of these friends were extremely high-powered and successful, everyone was equally down-to-earth and real. We were so relaxed and so happy just to be there.

Robert then drove me home and was a complete gentleman. It was pretty clear we both liked each other a lot—well, more than just a lot, as the air between us was practically electrified!—but we were both still too shy to make a move. He walked me to my door and thanked me for a lovely night, then kissed me sweetly on the cheek. I walked in the door and couldn't quite believe what had happened. I sat down on the sofa and kicked off my heels, giving Lola a cuddle as I replayed each and every amazing moment. Honestly, I felt like I was Debbie Reynolds in one of the MGM musicals I had watched with such awe when I was a child!

I realized my feelings were becoming overwhelming, but I also realized I had to be a professional and keep my cool. My plan was to tell him how I felt around week six or seven on the show, if we made it that far. I convinced myself that would be doable, but Robert thankfully soon blew that plan when, only a week later, he told me he had feelings for me.

When that wonderful moment happened, we were in Miami for one of Robert's car races. He loves racing and speed as much as he loves a business challenge and has competed in the North American Ferrari Challenge series for years. (He was voted rookie of the year in 2011!) Because Robert had already committed to this race, the *Dancing with the Stars* production team and I got to go with him, because we had to keep on rehearsing and filming these rehearsals for the upcoming show. Tough gig, I know! My friend Carson Kressley came with us because I knew I'd have a lot of downtime when Robert was on the track, and it would be great to have a friend in town to spend it with.

Because Carson knew me so well, he could tell how I was feeling. (Okay, so it was rather obvious . . . !) In fact, he was so worried I'd get my heart broken that he warned me about falling for Robert, who was newly single. Carson thought maybe it was more of a "showmance" or just a bit of fun, but after spending what felt like two seconds with Robert, Carson could tell how genuine, kind, and caring he really is. I think anyone who saw us together knew that we had something special and Carson was no different.

The day after we arrived, I went to watch Robert race. At first I thought how sexy he looked in his racing outfit and car, but when I saw him flying around the track with everyone I was so nervous for him. It was the real deal. They were serious out there; they were all intensely competitive and they all wanted to win. I was biting my nails when he edged into first place during the race, and some of the other drivers were trying to cut him off and overtake him on the corners. It came down to the wire and Robert finished in the top three.

I have no idea how he mustered the energy, but in between the two days of racing—I was exhausted just from watching him!—we squeezed in the rehearsals. And that's when I knew. I mean, I really *knew*. Yes, I had already been excited and interested and wanting more, but in Miami, seeing him in his element, doing something he loved with his friends, watching him on the track with his competitive spirit soaring as his car sped around the curves, that's when it truly clicked. I was so nervous for him and I was even more proud of his achievements. When the racing was done, I was nearly giddy over being able to spend time with Robert.

I knew I was falling madly and deeply in love with him. Falling hard. Harder than I'd ever fallen. And he was such a wonderful guy that I also knew it would be worth every second to give this relationship the shot it deserved.

When we got back to Los Angeles, we went right back to our usual rehearsal routine. We were in the thick of the show and loving every bit of it. My concerns about starting a romance while dancing on the show never came into it. We were very professional at the studio and Robert was the best student, working so hard and taking everything in. I think that's why he's so successful. When it's time to work he works!

Still, I think people watching us on the show could see a romance blossoming, and that's exactly what was happening. The main focus was, of course, the dancing, but we just loved spending time together and I guess it showed. Robert and I loved rehearsing and working toward this one common goal. And the more we worked together, the more I saw how much he just absolutely *loved* dancing. He was so proud of himself when he'd get the steps right. In fact, he was so enthusiastic about learning how to dance that his energy and determination gave me a newfound love for what I do. I really think we were bringing the best out in each other.

I also think that is part of what we respected so much about each other. I kept pinching myself as our romance was taking root on the show because I could not believe I was being paid to work with this awe-inspiring man. I had so much respect for him, and he had a lot of respect for me and what I was teaching him. I truly believe the best relationships are built on friendship and mutual respect, and that's what we had with each other.

In addition, we were both driven from a very early age to succeed at what we loved doing. We both made painful sacrifices to follow our dreams. We both got up in the morning and went back to work no matter how exhausted or stressed we were. We both knew what it was to basically live out of a suitcase because our work necessitated constant traveling. We both knew the toll that this kind of life could take on loving relationships. And we were both able to talk so freely with each other about all our past mistakes and what we'd learned from them.

The audience finally saw confirmation of our growing passion for each other during week seven, when we were dancing a contemporary dance to Jessie Ware's "Champagne Kisses." Robert suddenly kissed me on live television while we were in the middle of the dance. That particular moment just happened! During rehearsals, we had discussed whether or not the routine should have a kiss in it, but we just decided to go with it and either hug or kiss in that moment in the choreography. Clearly, we know how that turned out! After that, it was a bit harder to deny how much we cared about each other.

When we were eliminated I was sad because Robert had been working so hard, but mostly because I wouldn't be rehearsing with him every day anymore. But being off the show allowed us to date like normal people and go to a movie or dinner. I think that meeting Robert the way I did was incredible kismet, and it definitely fast-tracked our relationship. We were spending over six hours together every day and still had not had one moment where we were starting to get sick of each other. I truly believe we were meant to meet and I can't thank Deena Katz enough for pairing us together.

I look back on my life and failed relationships and everything makes sense now! It thrills me to no end to say that Robert is the most inspiring person I've ever met, with an enthusiasm for life and for learning new things that is amazingly infectious. Today, my relationship with Robert is even better than in our *Dancing with the Stars* days. We continue to adore, love, and respect each other. I wouldn't change a thing, as it all led me here, to this very moment. Who knows what the future holds, but I'm so excited about the next chapter.

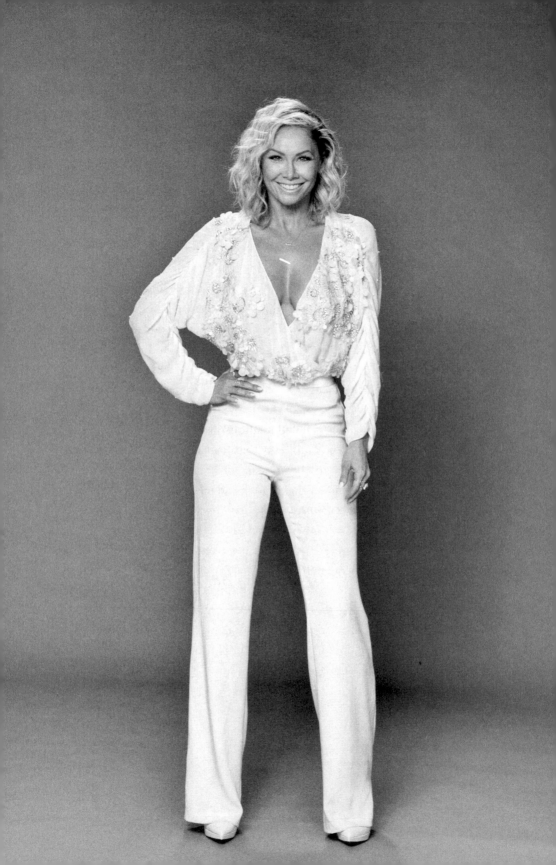

You've Made It!

We're old friends by now—you've made it!

By now, you've learned a lot about my approach to health, fitness, and nutrition. And you've also realized that the 5-6-7-8 Diet and Life Plan isn't only about how you look—it's about how you feel.

When I started writing this book, I wanted to share my years of dance experience with the world. I love coaching and helping motivate people to achieve their very best. I wanted women everywhere to understand that the goal isn't to be a size two with the toned, flat abs of a professional dancer. The goal is to move, to laugh, to love—and to feel a little bit better about yourself. I've had ups and downs along the way, just like everyone else. But, looking back over my life and accomplishments now makes me so gratified by how I've been able to overcome the obstacles and realize what truly makes me happy.

I know it's hard to watch TV or movies and idolize celebrities with very small waistlines and seemingly unrealistic appearances. I get it—because I do it, too! Remember, as a professional dancer I need to train for over six hours every day when I'm performing. I literally can't eat enough calories to keep the weight on. That might strike you as a good problem to have, but every dancer also knows that it's not realistic for day to day, especially when we aren't working. Now that my schedule has changed, I've had to adapt to a less active schedule, and the 5-6-7-8 Diet is a reflection of the food plan and workouts that I've incorporated into my daily routine to keep me fit, trim, full, and brimming with energy.

You're ready to take the next step. You've learned all about the benefits of consuming five lean proteins, six colors of the rainbow, seven anti-inflammatory properties, and eight glasses of water each day. You've also got an arsenal of workouts in your back pocket. Remember to start small. Do the core quickie, try some of the total body workouts, and then really get going and amp it up. Make a commitment to yourself to stick to your fourteen-day diet plan and your thirty-day workout calendar. Not only will you look better, but I promise you, you will feel better, too.

Don't forget to make sure you have a support system to help along the way. I know I wouldn't be here today without mine. Whether it's a loved one, a partner, a child, a friend—whoever it is, tell them about the changes you're making and encourage them to join you. Or, write down your goals as regular reminders. Remember my post-it notes with my favorite quotes? They're still all over my house. Tape them to your mirror in the bathroom so every morning you wake up and can say to yourself, "I can do this."

All the tools you need are within the pages of this book. My voice, as your very own personal coach, is reflected here. Know that this program doesn't stop after your fourteen-day weight loss program or your thirty-day workout calendar. It's a philosophy that you can follow, starting today, for the rest of your life. Whatever your journey may be, use this plan to help fuel your success.

Can't resist doing it one last time . . . and a five, six, seven, eight!

With love,
Kym

Acknowledgments

A project like this doesn't come together without the love and support of so many. You've all touched my life in such unique ways and I'm grateful for your help in bringing my vision to life.

To my mum, Barbara Johnson: I could not do any of this without you. Thank you for our daily calls. Sometimes it's just to say hi, but it means the world. Thank you for all the encouragement, love, and support. You've supported me through all the ups and downs and I'm lucky to have you as my best friend.

To my father, Eddie Johnson: Thank you for all the props you made me so I could perform with nothing but the best. Thank you for always driving me to practice and for the constant encouragement and love.

To Robert: My life changed when I met you. You inspire me every day to pursue my dreams. You encouraged me to write this book, and I'm so grateful for your love and support. You make me want to be the best person I can be and I love you.

To Karen Moline, my writing partner in crime: I couldn't have done this without you. Your energy, enthusiasm, and passion for this project really brought my vision to life. Thank you for being my sounding board and supporting this book every step of the way. I'm so proud of what we've done together.

To Judith Regan and the incredible team at Regan Arts: Max, Richard, Nancy, and Lynne. I will never forget the day I met you in your office in NYC. I was excited and nervous to pitch my book idea to you. I was surprised at how enthusiastic you were about it. Judith, you are a genius and know how to get the most out of people. Thank you for having faith in me and for making this experience so enjoyable. You've brought this book to life and I've appreciated your expertise, creative support, and guidance every step of the way.

To Rachel Tonick: You're such a genius and it's incredible to see your success with FitLife Productions. Thank you for seeing the potential in my fitness program and helping me bring it to life in 5-6-7-8 Fitness. You put in the time with me in the dance studio to refine the movements and photos that will bring this program to life for so many incredible women around the world. My glutes are still in pain from all the lunges we did together!!

To Jennifer Cassetta: You captured my diet philosophy in such a simple way. We created 5-6-7-8 to make it easy to remember how to incorporate lean proteins, all the colors of the rainbow, and anti-inflammatory properties into your diet each day—and you just got it! Thank you for helping make this program so healthy and delicious. Be sure to visit JenniferCassetta.com to check out some of Jen's own recipes and workouts.

To Joel Gotler and Murray Weiss: Thank you for believing in me and my passion to bring this book to life. You brought me to Judith and the team at Regan Arts, and I'm so appreciative of your support.

To Erin McLean: I couldn't have done this without you. You have been the driving force for this book from day one. You are so inspiring to me—such an incredible woman with great vision and passion for everything you do. You have been there from the initial meetings in New York City to the exciting call telling me I actually had a book deal! Your constant love, support, and friendship through this has been incredible. I'm going to miss our daily FaceTime status updates. I think we will just have to get started on book number two!

To Kaleigh Tait: You are one talented lady! Thanks for bringing my branding vision for 5-6-7-8 Fitness to life in this book and on my website.

To my dear friend Glenn Nutley: Thank you for taking so many of the photos in this book that help bring *5-6-7-8* Fitness to life. Most of all, thanks for being the best friend to me. I've known you my whole life. We've been through so many ups and downs together, and you've been there through everything. You are so incredibly talented and I adore you. Please check out Glenn's website to see just how amazing he is: GlennNutley.com.

To Lesley Bryce: It was such a pleasure to meet you through this process and I love how all the workout poses turned out. Thank you for capturing the movement of the exercises so well.

To Kath, Sara, and Crystal: Thanks to my ultimate glam team! Kath, thank you for the incredible hair and makeup you do. You are such an incredible energy to be around! Sara, thank you for all the looks you came up with for me on *Dancing with the Stars* and thank you for doing my makeup for the photos in this book. You are gorgeous inside and out. Crystal, thank you for doing such amazing hair for the book's photos. You are so talented and can literally do anything. You make me laugh and I love your spirit!

To my *Dancing with the Stars* family, Joe Sunker, Deena Katz, Rob Wade, and Michael Brooks: Thank you for giving me my start on *Dancing with the Stars*. Rob, I will never forget the phone call I received in Australia telling me you wanted me in LA in a week to start on the show. Being a part of *DWTS* is so much more than a job. As cheesy as it sounds it's really one big family. I have loved every second of being on the show and it has opened so many doors and brought such incredible opportunities my way. I'm forever grateful. I'd also like to take this moment to thank the incredible pros, crew, production team, glam squads, and of course contestants on *Dancing with the Stars* over the past twenty-one seasons. (Twenty-one seasons? Incredible.) It's such an honor and a blessing to be part of this show.

To the stunning Florence Henderson (everyone's favorite mom): Thank you for your friendship and motherly advice. I loved being on *Dancing with the Stars* with you but love how our friendship has developed even more. You are always so positive, happy, and fun to be around. I just adore you. Thanks for sharing your yummy recipes and advice in this book.

To the lovely Cheryl Burke: You were the first one to talk to me when I was the new girl on set. Thank you for being such a great friend and for contributing some of your health and fitness philosophy to this book.

To the charismatic Joey Fatone: Thank you for being you! You are one of the funniest people I know with the biggest heart, and you would do anything for anyone. We may have come in second and not received the Mirror Ball (and you never let me forget it), but I got you as a lifelong friend! Thanks for sharing your experiences and advice for this book.